FOREWORD

WE live in a litigious society — in which the psychiatrist may often be called upon to participate in various court proceedings. What goes on in his consulting room, or what he has learned throughout his professional life, is now easily and often brought to witness in a courtroom. Beyond his training in physical medicine and human behavior, today's psychiatrist may often need to be versed in the rules of law.

Psychiatry and Law by Ralph Slovenko, LL.B., Ph.D., was distinguished by receiving the Guttmacher Award for outstanding scientific writing.

Lederle Laboratories is proud to be able to bring you this important and informative book, in its entirety, in four volumes. The volumes will be presented to you during the course of the year at regular intervals.

As the developer and producer of LOXITANE® Loxapine Succinate and LOXITANE® C Loxapine Hydrochloride, Lederle Laboratories has demonstrated its continued commitment to developing better products for better patient care. Lederle Laboratories is confident that Dr. Slovenko's book will be as valuable in your reference library as will be LOXITANE in your armamentarium of effective drugs.

PSYCHIATRY AND LAW

RALPH SLOVENKO, LL.B., Ph.D.

Professor of Law and Psychiatry
Wayne State University School of Law
Detroit, Michigan

Little, Brown and Company
Boston

Published December 1973

Copyright © 1973 by Little, Brown and Co. (Inc.)

First Edition
Second Printing

Library of Congress catalog card No. 73-331

ISBN 0-316-79868-1

Printed in the United States of America

In Memory of My Father

PREFACE

ONCE an arcane subject matter, the interplay of psychiatry and law since about 1960 has emerged from the elective seminar room of the university to become a topic of national prominence. It now has a high visibility profile. Several factors account for this development.

First of all, an increased population concentrated in urban areas makes more important the formalized relationships among people as expressed in law. With expanding governmental programs, the legal machinery becomes especially important since all these programs are mediated through the law. As psychiatry, like law, is a specialty directly concerned with the appropriate regulation of human behavior, the psychiatrist can contribute to the substantive areas of the programs and assist in determining the methods by which these programs will be implemented.

In this time of unparalleled violence and spoliation of the environment, the failure of psychiatry to speak out on social planning would be not only irresponsible but tragic. The public confidence in psychiatry would grow in direct proportion to the profession's ability to deal with a multiplicity of causes—physical, emotional, environmental—that may figure in any case, even though this requires a break from orthodoxy. In dealing with any behavior the following points are always to be considered: What does the behavior mean for the individual? What does it reveal about his emotional condition? What does it reveal about the family from which he comes? What does it reveal about the community from which he comes? And what changes should take place in the individual, the family, and the community?

A second factor contributing to the developing interaction of psychiatry and law is that psychiatry has taken over many functions of religion, which at one time highly influenced the law. Many legal principles that had their source in religion are now supplied by psychiatry. Psychiatry is having profound effects on the very meaning of life. Many individuals who previously consulted with a clergyman now take their problems to a psychotherapist. Many who belonged to a church group for social purposes now join a therapy group. Psychiatric explanations have replaced religious prohibitions in regard to sexual behavior, drinking, and gambling. Psychiatric concepts now prevail in the realm of abortion and birth control and are being used to establish what is or is not obscene and pornographic.

Third, emphasis in handling offenders is currently placed on concepts of rehabilitation rather than on those of revenge and retribution. Rehabilitative programs demand psychiatric contributions; but this demand has been and continues to be resisted by many psychiatrists. Psychiatry as a profession has essentially abdicated its role in the handling of offenders. Psychiatric services are essentially unavailable in prison. At the same time those few psychiatrists who see a role for their expertise in this area find that prison milieu thwarts their efficacy, or that they have to do battle with groups who feel that psychiatry is trespassing when it tries to offer its contributions.

Fourth, the practice of psychiatry is gradually shifting. Many more young people are seeing psychiatrists. There are relatively more people with antisocial and behavioral problems than with subjective neurotic symptomatology and classical psychosis in the form of dementia praecox. At the same time, under the *parens patriae* doctrine, the state is viewed as having the duty to intervene in the lives of all minors who might become community problems.

Fifth, while lawyers are generally no more interested than psychiatrists in dealing with criminal offenders or public mental-hospital patients, there has been a substantial increase in lawyer involvement and litigation in this area, essentially due to the financial support by public, private, and charitable organizations. Perhaps indicative of this recently developed interest of the legal profession in problems of law as related to mental disorder is the inclusion for the first time of a special topic, *Mental Health,* in the *Sixth Decennial Digest,* the digest of court cases. *Mental Health Court Digest,* a monthly summary of reported state and federal court decisions relating to mental health, is prepared especially for mental health agencies and personnel.

Sixth, during the past decade a substantial body of literature as well as caselaw on psychiatry and law has developed. In particular, the decisions of Chief Judge David L. Bazelon of the District of Columbia Circuit Court of Appeals, which figure prominently in any collection of cases, and the writings (available in paperback) of Dr. Karl A. Menninger and of Dr. Thomas S. Szasz have stimulated discussion regarding the role of the psychiatrist in the legal process. Their untraditional and pioneering views are provocative and have reached a wide audience, including television viewers. For many students, it is Szasz's writings which prompt registration in law-psychiatry courses. One might take issue with these writings, but they will certainly be found interesting.

Seventh, there has developed during recent years a number of extended

programs of study and research and a number of professional organizations in law and the behavioral sciences. Paralleling the broadening of
the scope of psychiatric residency training programs to include community problems, concern about curriculum relevance has prompted law
schools to seek breadth and depth in legal education. Foundations have
made substantial grants to a number of law schools to establish inter-
disciplinary teaching and research in law and the behavioral sciences.
The recently formed American Academy of Psychiatry and the Law
(AAPL) and the American Psychology-Law Society (AP-LS) are rapidly
growing in membership. The AAPL, founded in late 1969 by a group of
15 teachers in law and psychiatry, now has a membership, limited to psychiatrists, of about 250. The AP-LS, organized at the 1968 annual meeting of the American Psychological Association, includes lawyers and law
professors in its membership of over 300. The International Academy of
Forensic Psychology, founded in 1968, has membership in 14 countries
and approximately 250 members, including psychologists, psychiatrists,
social workers, correctional workers, attorneys, judges, and police officers.
In addition, the American College of Legal Medicine, founded in 1955
primarily as an organization for persons who hold degrees in both law
and medicine, now has approximately 100 Fellows. The American Academy of Forensic Sciences, founded in 1948, has a membership of approximately 900 composed of physicians who are specialists in forensic pathology, forensic psychiatry, and other forensic medical areas. There is also
the Association for Psychiatric Treatment of Offenders (APTO) and the
Medical Correctional Association. There are now, apart from a number
of newsletters, several specialized journals—the *Journal of Psychiatry and
Law, Bulletin of Psychiatry and the Law, Journal of Forensic Psychology,
Journal of Forensic Sciences, International Journal of Offender Therapy,*
and *Corrective Psychiatry and Journal of Social Therapy.* Many law reviews published by law schools present symposia or feature articles on
law and psychiatry. As a by-product, these activities stir up interest outside the professional circle.

An eighth factor of significance is that increased familiarity of judges
and lawyers with psychiatry has resulted in large numbers of referrals to
psychiatric agencies from both civil and criminal cases. The traditional
concepts of the criminal law are being questioned, and it appears quite
likely, both on theoretical and logistical grounds, that differences between civil commitment for involuntary treatment and criminal commitment for rehabilitation will gradually diminish. Society may end up with
two kinds of institutions: the mental hospital for treatment on a voluntary

basis and the correctional institution for the involuntary treatment or confinement of those who are bothersome to society.

Assuming that this evaluation trend is correct, the burden on the psychiatric community will materially increase. There are now approximately 240,000 inmates in state and federal prisons and well over one million inmates in county jails, a large majority of whom are disturbed mentally. As this tremendous load is added to the task of the "helping professions," additional personnel must be employed in nontraditional ways. Some universities, anticipating this growing need, have already developed training programs in departments of social work, sociology, and police science.

One segment of society is impatient with psychiatry for moving so slowly into areas which so obviously require the profession's knowledge and expertise; other segments of society, however, are either apathetic or openly hostile, viewing the introduction of any psychiatric concepts into the administration of the law as a force which will weaken the fabric of society. Most members of the legal profession share the mixed values of the community at large, but a number of leaders in the profession press for additional services from psychiatry which would make possible increased referral of cases and the participation of psychiatrists in the courts.

Law and psychiatry are now challenged in their treatment of offenders and mentally disordered persons. Judge Bazelon, at a conference in 1965 of the American Psychiatric Association on planning comprehensive community mental health services, charged that psychiatry has been largely indifferent to the moral dilemma that the law raises in the courtroom. In the new as well as old mental health facilities, psychiatry discourages referral of offenders by arguments like *"these people* are untreatable . . . don't keep appointments," etc. Judge Bazelon noted that there may be an element of truth in the objections, but they are also devices by which psychiatrists make life easier for themselves and abdicate their social responsibility. Professional life can be much easier when dealing with the small problems of the rich than with the large but financially unrewarding problems of the poor.

Until now, the community has thought only in terms of piecemeal solutions to such problems as crime and delinquency, obscenity, addiction, malingering, divorce, and child custody; when psychiatry was acknowledged it was viewed as being applicable only to segments of the problems. What psychiatry has learned from the intensive care of a few has not been applied to the problems that involve many. It is roughly analogous to treating the pallor of disseminated malignancy with a sun-lamp. The community will see what psychiatry may, in fact, have to offer to the solution of such problems only when adequately trained psychiatrists offer a full range of services to the individual involved, to the institutions and their staffs, and to the community at large. The objection that social and political issues are beyond the scope of the psychiatrist's skills or his ability to do something useful about them usually assumes a medical model of a patient, or it constitutes an abdication of responsibility. Not to go beyond the immediate concerns of daily work is to ignore the fundamental role played by institutions in shaping behavior. If we want less imperfect human beings, the American founding fathers said, the place to begin is by building a less imperfect society.

In an industrial society the sphere in which the law operates is quite extensive: it determines the status of individuals and the existing order of social relations; it regulates property relations, the measure and forms of distribution of labor and its products; it fixes the forms of administration and the constitutional system; it determines the activity of the state mechanism and lays down the measures for combating encroachments on the state system. With the decline in the force and influence of private sources of moral and social obligations, the law has played an increasing role in regulating the economy, in controlling or facilitating technology, in ordering race relations, and in regulating morality and the environment.

As a discipline, the law is divided into a number of categories, including crimes, torts, contracts, property, and domestic relations. Psychiatry appears as a subtopic under these subdivisions, as illustrated in the following examples. A *mens rea*, i.e., a guilty mind, is an essential element in the criminal law. Much of the law of torts rests upon the intent or negligence of the individual sought to be found liable. One of the general theories of the law of contracts is that the contracting parties must have a "meeting of the minds." The validity of testamentary disposition of property is based on the mental competency of the testator at the time of the execution of the will.

These are some of the areas in which psychiatry has played a role in law. Conversely, the law has played a role in psychiatry, as illustrated by the regulation of psychiatric practice and hospital procedures.

The interface of psychiatry and law is commonly termed *forensic psychiatry*, *legal psychiatry*, or the new and broader phrase *social-legal psy-*

chiatry, which includes all aspects of psychiatry in close and significant contact with the law. The interface area, which is related in these pages, includes problems in the psychiatric aspects of criminal responsibility, disposition of offenders, addiction to alcohol and drugs, commitment procedures and rights of the mentally ill, civil competency, personal injury evaluation, marriage and divorce, custody of children, abortion, malpractice litigation, regulation of psychiatric practice, psychiatric testimony in courts or before legislative bodies, and confidentiality of communications.

The interface of psychiatry and the criminal law is, in part at least, already developed or in the process of development. The other phases of law-psychiatry have lagged behind. In virtually all areas, including the criminal, the experts who are called upon to give opinions are dissatisfied with lawyers, the law, and the conditions under which they must assist in the administration of justice. The lawyers and the courts are equally dissatisfied with the experts.

This volume is designed to serve three principal purposes. First, it is intended to serve as a course textbook for psychiatric residents and law students, and as a basic reference source for the psychiatrist or lawyer who is only occasionally confronted with problems in law and psychiatry. Secondly, it is designed to assist those practitioners who regularly work in this area by suggesting new approaches and by providing material to assist them in preparing and documenting their cases. Thirdly, it is intended to provide a critical exposition of many of the practices and basic premises of the terrain of law and psychiatry.

Acknowledgments

I cannot hope to acknowledge my debt to all the people who have influenced the ideas that appear in this book. I do, though, first want to pay homage to my father, who died suddenly while this book was being prepared. My interest in psychiatry probably began on that day of my boyhood when my father gave me as one of my first books, Freud's *Moses and Monotheism*. Years later my friend, Dr. Gene L. Usdin, stimulated my interest in psychiatry when I was a professor of law at Tulane University, and at the invitation of Dr. Robert G. Heath, Chairman of the Department of Psychiatry and Neurology at Tulane, I was permitted, although not a medical-school graduate, to undertake the three-year-residency training program in psychiatry with a view to working in the law-psychiatry field. I am grateful to Dr. Heath and colleagues for this unique opportunity, and for an educational experience that remains the most exciting of my life. I owe thanks to Ray Forrester, then Dean of the Tulane Law School, who helped make it possible.

I was subsequently, for over three years, on the staff of the Menninger Foundation, on a joint appointment with the University of Kansas School of Law, and I am grateful to Dr. Karl A. Menninger and colleagues for another stimulating experience. Dr. Karl at the time was writing his book, *The Crime of Punishment*, and we had many interesting discussions which influenced my ideas. I also want to express my appreciation to James K. Logan, then Dean of the Kansas Law School, and colleagues for cosponsoring my joint appointment.

As I became increasingly involved in the world of psychiatry, I learned much that was new to me from friends and colleagues, most particularly Drs. Robert G. Heath, Arthur Epstein, Edward H. Knight, James A. Knight, Harold I. Lief, Elliot D. Luby, Karl A. Menninger, Herbert C. Modlin, Edward C. Norman, Cyril Phillips, Joseph Satten, C. B. Scrignar, Frank Silva, William C. Super, Karl Targownik, and Gene L. Usdin.

While some parts of this book were prepared before my joining the faculty of the Wayne State University School of Law, it was mainly done there. I wish to express my thanks to the law library staff for meeting my endless requests for materials with gracious and dedicated efforts; I am grateful to Dean Charles W. Joiner and colleagues for a delightful atmosphere. I am most thankful to Mr. Vernon P. Saper and Mrs. Susan W. Bagwell who, each in their third year of law study, served admirably as my research assistants. I am especially thankful to Mrs. Phyllis Wright and Miss Susan Battersby for their advisory and secretarial assistance. They were superb.

I thank Judge Luther A. Alverson of the Atlanta Superior Court, Dr. Peter Hartocollis of the Menninger Foundation, and Dr. Richard L. Jenkins of the University of Iowa for studying the entire manuscript and offering valuable suggestions.

Ralph Slovenko

CONTENTS

Between the idea
And the reality

. . . .

Falls the Shadow

—T. S. ELIOT

I. THE PSYCHIATRIST AND PROOF AT LAW

1. EVIDENCE IN THE JUDICIAL PROCESS

AT first sight, few things seem further apart than the domains of law and games, for one seems solemn and the other playful, but there are many common elements. The Greek word *agonia* referred to any kind of contest or conflict, and also meant mental anguish. In considerable measure, the judicial process and the rules on evidence find explanation in the theory of games that people play. This relationship is currently drawing much attention in the psychological and social sciences and has prompted Abraham Goldstein, Dean of the Yale Law School, to observe, "Anyone familiar with games theory and with the growing literature on role playing will readily see their analogue in the adversary system."

John Huizinga, a Dutch historian, in a brilliant book called *Homo Ludens* (1944), describes the play element in culture and points out the affinity between law and play. In biological terms, man is usually called *Homo sapiens:* man (genus) the intelligent (species), a singularly unconvincing description. Later man has been called *Homo faber,* meaning "man the tool-maker and -user." Huizinga suggests that man might be called *Homo ludens,* the human being that plays. (*Homo ludens* means "man while he is [for a little time] playing"; the term actually needed is *Homo lusor,* "man as a sportsman, a lover of play [permanently].") *Ludo, ergo sum;* I play, therefore I am. The truly *ludic* is play that brings about autonomous discipline; the *ludicrous* is games-playing social behavior that is obedient to a narrow set of rules.

Twenty years later, Dr. Eric Berne, in *Games People Play* (1964), described the commonplace interpersonal pattern or social disturbance created to gain some secret relief or satisfaction as a game. Berne points out that people tend to live their lives by consistently playing out certain "games" in their interpersonal relationships, which they play for a variety of reasons: to avoid confronting reality, to deal with helplessness, to conceal ulterior motives, to rationalize their activities, or to avoid actual participation. These games—if they are not destructive—are both desirable and necessary. The "courtroom game" in its everyday form, Berne says, is easily observed among children as a three-handed game between two siblings and a parent:

"Mommie, she took my candy away."

"Yes, but he took my doll, and before that he was hitting me, and anyway we both promised to share our candy."

In his thesaurus of games, Berne offers examples which strike many a familiar chord.[1] The childhood prototype of cops and robbers is hide-and-seek, in which the essential element is the chagrin at being found. (The game is now called "cops and robbers and lawyers and Supreme Court.") Among older children, one who finds an insoluble hiding place is regarded as not being a good sport, since he has spoiled the game. It is also deemed unsportsmanlike conduct for the police to hide behind plain clothes or to entrap suspects. In childhood, deception is aggravating.

The adversary method of trial, or "gamesmanship under the gavel," is well suited to the popular Anglo-American conditioning to games. The phrase *sporting theory of justice* is an apt description of their judicial process. The concept is not popular everywhere; the games that people play depend upon their families and society as a whole. Consider, for example, the observation of Luigi Barzini, who is responsible for the following: "Many rules of 'fair play' appear to the Italians as a joke. Such as the English formula, 'Do not hit a fallen enemy'! . . . When would it be better and more advantageous to hit him?"

In play a child achieves mastery over helplessness. Play is the child's work; recreation is indeed re-creation. In the re-creation of a traumatic event, he turns a passive experience in which he has been a victim into one in which he is in charge. Thus, upon coming home, a child who has had a frightening experience at the dentist's may do dental work on his pet. A child who has been in the hospital may want to play with bandaged dolls, miniature intravenous poles, and toy beds. Assuming the active role, the child masters the experience psychically. Another illustration is ring-around-the-rosy, a game of joining hands, forming a circle of life, which began in medieval Europe to mock the peril of the black death.

The same psychodynamic prevails in adults. In an observation now famous, Nietzsche remarked that hidden in every man is a child who wants to play. Freud showed in detail the ways in which the infantile past survives in the adult. Berne in his work on Transactional Analysis points out that every person is actually three—child, adult, and parent; at any given time, a person's ego state may be that of a child, adult, or parent. There is a popular saying, "People don't really grow up, they just play with bigger toys." Grown men are driven by essentially the same forces as children, and the way that men deal with these forces is permeated and affected by the experiences of their childhoods. *Monopoly*, a board game in which real estate and properties are bought and traded for large sums of money, was created by an unemployed salesman during the economic depression of the 1930s. Active mastery of the reality of economic helplessness was not possible for most people during this period, but passive mastery through the game fantasy of enormous compensatory wealth and power was possible. The game struck a responsive chord in the universal anxiety of the times.

A recurrence of childlike magic is to be expected in conditions of intense anxiety or preoccupation with a particular desire. To say that an adult is acting childishly has the flavor of an insult, but to behave in a childlike manner in certain adult contexts may be the very best way of coping with a situation.

Like the individual, society sutures itself by re-creating in a trial an event that has disturbed its peace. In doing so, society asserts its mastery. A trial resolves conflict and serves to educate, as does play. As in play, adherence to the rules set out in law contributes to the formation of individual conscience.

The judicial process was initially a contest and has always been subject to restrictive rules which set the lawsuit squarely in the domain of orderly, antithetical play. Pronouncement of justice takes place in a court, in a kind of sacred circle, a place set off from the ordinary world. The ambience of the theater envelops the proceeding. Like show business, the law makes use of certain properties. Judges don robes and sometimes wigs. Scenery, too, is as important to a legal drama as it is to the theatrical play. The courtroom production begins with the court crier's "Oyez," announcing the coming of the judge.

When the judge tours or plays in the provinces, he is said to go on "circuit." When the judge came to town, on his circuit, the cry went out, "Here comes the judge!" and people all assembled. Apart from going to church, attending a trial was formerly the big event in the lives of the people.

Traditionally, a trial has been regarded as a type of drama and is preeminently a theatrical form. The trial, like the classical form of the drama, is always a contest between protagonist and antagonist, the resolution of the play being comparable to the verdict on the action. A very early account in history of a trial comes from the drama, *The Eumenides*, of Aeschylus' trilogy, the *Oresteia*. Like the old morality play, the trial presents in dramatic fashion the conflicting moral values of the community. Thurman Arnold says that both civil and criminal trials perform this function, but since the criminal law is the buttress of morality, the criminal process has more important emotional impact upon society.[2] Thus, like the morality play, the criminal trial seeks to vindicate moral values. The struggle features the universal agony of morality or the passionate tension between good and evil.[3]

The art of acting is as necessary in a trial as in a play or drama. Advocates like Clarence Darrow have been popular favorites, regarded by the public with much the same affection as that extended to athletes and actors. Advocates have always trained themselves to give histrionic displays in the legal drama in which they were engaged. Cicero studied the performances of Aesopus and Roscius, the theatrical stars of his day. In Athens every man acted as his own lawyer, but the profession of speech writer developed to help those who were inept. The Ionian Sophists, who hired philosophers to defend disputes in court and engaged in spectacular exercises of logic, were ridiculed by Socrates, who (through Plato) made out of his trial a very entertaining play.

The importance of advocacy is exemplified in the lifetime record of Texas attorney Percy Foreman—700 wins against one loss. It was clearly not the rightness of the client's case that won all these decisions in his favor. Rather, this score results from Foreman's ability to make black look white. (In one case, he threatened to reveal the "truth" if a $⅓-million fee were not paid.) One columnist put it thus: "Foreman, like most successful trial lawyers, often plays the ham, diverting the minds of the jury from whatever the prosecution may be trying to prove."[4]

Much "truth" is accepted through faith. Without denying or affirming its validity, there is the belief of a virgin birth and of heaven and hell. The phrase *seeing is believing* may be turned around—*believing is seeing*. Psychological testing—for example, Rorschach's ink-blot test and Murray's thematic apperception test—recognizes that the individual projects himself into his receptive and assertive relations with the world. Freud pointed out how much we shape our thoughts and ideas to suit our moods and needs.

A person would rather have one good soul-satisfying emotion than a dozen facts. "Reason against passion!" Einstein wrote. "The latter always wins if there's any struggle at all. . . ." The solemn ceremony of the trial, the prescribed formalities, the stereotyped patterns of speech, the long deliberations and sifting of evidence are designed to control emotions and to allow "sovereign reason" to prevail. They form a protective screen, much like the compulsive ceremonials of the neurotic, in trying to keep emotions under control. An emotion, which is a passion, ceases to be a passion, Spinoza said, when we form a clear and distinct idea of it. Although the trial lawyer relies on histrionics, the judge or jury often sense that his exclamatory words—"This is outrageous," "I could not object more"—do not really reflect his underlying feelings. In any event, the thespian activities of the advocates aside, everything in the judicial process is directed to the elimination of emotions. The relationship of judge or jury and litigant is institutionalized in an attempt to exclude the many irrelevancies which spring from human frailty.

In the view of many, a trial is expected to establish the truth and to explain an event. A common assumption is that a trial, if fairly conducted, will provide complete information to the public about an event of concern to it. After all, a witness does swear "to tell the truth, the whole truth, and nothing but the truth." Thus, when James Earl Ray entered a plea of guilty to the murder of Martin Luther King, there was an outcry in the press that the public was being denied the facts of the assassination. One news editor complained, "Too many questions remain unanswered . . . the court did not seek the answers. It was no search for truth. It was no search at all."[5]

A trial, however, is not an investigative but essentially a demonstrative proceeding, which, according to predetermined norms and a particular mode of proof, evaluates only the evidence brought forth by the parties. It is not expected that a trial, however fair, will produce all the evidence that exists. Moreover, however important its public function, a trial is not obligatory; the guilty plea, or plea bargaining, is a legal prerogative of the accused. Quite often, both society and the defendant are better served by the less expensive, expeditious plea-bargaining process than they are by a trial.[6]

The law's method of inquiry, while it attempts to be dispassionate, differs substantially from the scientific inquiry. The functions and aims of the two, after all, are quite different. There are differences between law and science in intellectual objectives as well as emotional and attitudinal differences. The fundamental aim of law is justice while that of science is knowledge or truth. Results in law are primarily practical, and only secondarily theoretical.[7]

The researcher in experimental work sets up a number of competing hypotheses to be tested one by one. A legal decision-maker may do this to a certain point, but ultimately he must decide in favor of a single version. Victory (winning as the lawyers put it) is for one party *or* the other, as on the playing field; and the outcome of a case is often unpredictable. The chancery court is commonly referred to as the "chances court."

There are many areas in which the legal and the scientific inquiries can be compared and differences noted. Some include:

1. A lawsuit is not an abstract search for truth, but a proceeding to settle a controversy between two or more persons without physical conflict. The primary purpose of each case is to resolve an individual controversy rather than to contribute to the development of a general theory. The court does not entertain moot controversies. The work of science, on the other hand, is a corporate effort which attempts to ascertain empirical relationships through the examination of repeated instances and has for its purpose the growth of a body of general principles.[8]

2. The fact-finding processes of science and of law differ in methods used to secure and test data. The scientist selects facts with a view to supporting or testing hypotheses. In law, evidence is gathered by mutually antagonistic parties. The lawyers are involved as partisans interested in the outcome of the case. Loyalty to client comes before loyalty to truth. In the adversary process the court, which undertakes no investigation, adjudicates or decides between the competing claims, with each side attempting to develop the evidence that is helpful to its side and to play down or exclude evidence harmful to it. The law has policy reasons for this practice, which do not concern the scientist. As in any debate, out of the friction a type of truth may emerge.

3. The legal system's method of screening data—the rules of evidence —was developed and persists for reasons that pertain uniquely to the legal craft. Under the adversary system the trial judge considers only those objections which the attorneys urge; he is not required to search for other objections which have not been asserted. The rules of admission and exclusion of evidence are not self-operative. Counsel for the litigants must be alert to obtain the benefits of the rules and to employ recognized methods to exclude improper evidence, as well as to secure the admission of acceptable evidence. A party is bound by the objections which he makes to the evidence offered in the trial and is regarded as having waived all objections other than those specifically asserted. If an objection is not urged, evidence is admitted for whatever effect it may have in the solution of the fact issues.

4. Much evidence may be rejected in a court of law, even though in other disciplines it is considered substantial enough from which to draw inferences. The law may suppress evidence even though it clearly estab-

lishes an accused's guilt, as when, for example, an overzealous law-enforcement officer fails to comply with the technical requirements for a search warrant. The objective is to educate policemen to respect the rights of a suspect, although as a by-product it allows guilty men to go free. Further, on the basis of evidentiary rules, information may be withheld on the grounds of privileged communication. Science is not bound by such considerations and may utilize evidence from any source, however indirect.

5. The court is hampered by limitations of time and place. In the "heat and hurry" of the trial, a solution may leave a good deal to be desired. The courts say, "A defendant is entitled to a fair trial but not a perfect one." Aristotle said centuries ago: "We must not look for the same degree of accuracy in all subjects; we must be content in each class of subjects with accuracy of such kind as the subject matter allows." Dean John Wigmore observed, "A scientist can wait till he finds the data he wants; and he can use past, present, and future data; and he can go anywhere to get them. . . . But a judicial trial must be held at a fixed time and place, and the decision must be then made, once for all."[9]

6. The law's method of arriving at a result is often purposely nonscientific or dependent upon a nonprofessional assessment. However able a judge may be, he is usually no expert on the subject matter before him. Frequently, the results or verdicts are announced as the general, flat, unexplained decision of untrained minds—the jury—purposely selected for their lack of training. In its earliest form, the jury, drawn from the local community, relied on its own knowledge of the facts, however obtained. Witnesses as we know them today were rarely called; the jurors themselves were both witnesses and judge. In slow steps evolved the present but totally different method of trial by jury, which well may be less effective as a factfinder.

7. Science is not concerned with values, but only with formal relationships between observable events. Results in science are based on measurement and are obtained mathematically. Results in law, on the other hand, are influenced but not ruled by hard data or hard facts. Scientific evidence, no matter how reliable, is not conclusive and binding on the court. Justice incorporates social needs as well as scientific accuracy, but neither to the exclusion of the other. In the case most often cited by those who advocate taking away from the jury the right to reject scientific evidence, Charlie Chaplin in 1946 was held to be the father of Joan Berry's child notwithstanding blood-grouping tests excluding him. In paternity cases generally, a desire to legitimize the child or to find a

financially responsible person to care for the child has more meaning for the court than a blood test. This consideration was not standing alone in the *Chaplin* case, as moral considerations were also present. Other evidence showed that Chaplin and Berry had been living together in an illicit relationship. Although his sperm did not happen to meet with her egg, the jury in its concern for the welfare of the child felt that he should bear the responsibility. (Another jury shortly before, notwithstanding the cold-war climate of the time, acquitted Chaplin of a criminal charge under the Mann Act, which prohibits the transporting of women from one state to another for prostitution.) Another dramatic illustration of values in the decision-making process is the case of Angela Davis. A number of psychologists assisted defense attorneys in determining traits that would indicate whether or not a juror was likely to acquit. One implication of an acquittal was to defuse local and foreign militant propaganda.

8. The element of subjectivity is vastly greater in law or psychiatry than in the natural sciences, but this is not to say that fantasies or dreams do not play a role in science, as may be illustrated by the theories of scientists inspired by their dreams. In evaluating human behavior, though, one must constantly be making inferences, and it is precisely in making these inferences that judge or jury or psychiatrist can go astray. In law or psychiatry, dreams or fantasies may furnish clues as to the real facts. In talking with a criminal defendant about his dreams and fantasies, it may, or may not, become obvious that he was expecting an assault and was acting in self-defense. In talking with an injured person about his dreams, it may become obvious that he is either malingering or suffering a traumatic neurosis. In an unusual but interesting custody case, it was argued that one spouse should not have any form of visitation rights, based upon inferences drawn from his dream diary in which a number of sex dreams were recorded.[10] To stave off his son's attempt to have him declared mentally incompetent to manage his affairs, Sophocles (when about ninety years old) defended himself by reading passages from his latest play, *Oedipus at Colonus*, which he had just written.

9. Procedure—which is basically a form of Emily Post etiquette—is more important in law than in science. The content or substantive issues of the law are often resolved indirectly via questions of procedure. The name of the game, lawyers say, is *procedure*. To spit against the wind is to spit in one's own face, and to approach the real issue directly in law is to do just about the same.

10. Law and psychiatry may be called sciences of human behavior,

but the practice of lawyering or psychotherapy is an art. Foreman's score has already been mentioned. To achieve justice in the form of a favorable decision, attorneys resort to various tactics to overcome the element of chance. Sporting theory or no, there is something of Machiavelli in it. Like the play of bridge hands, what may be good tactics in one case may be quite unsuitable in another. One tactic which is followed consistently, however, concerns the dialogue of a trial, technically called *evidence*. Like the dialogue of a play, it is rarely a matter of improvisation. The attorney, although he does not write parts for his witnesses, rehearses them carefully in their proofs to see that they are letter perfect. Like Hamlet, he strongly urges them to "speak no more than is set down for them." One golden rule of advocacy is, "Never ask a question unless you know the answer." Sometimes, however, due to the pressure of work, the attorney is forced to go to a trial unprepared, a practice called "shooting from the hip," which often will result in improvised evidence.

11. A trial is basically a tribal ceremony. Julian Barry's Broadway play, *Lenny*, based on the prosecution of Lenny Bruce for obscenity, depicts the trial as a tribal development, complete with drums, chants, and a ritual of sacrifice. The costumes, though they seem to imply a sort of semi-caveman–tribal situation, are of no specific region. Like any trial, the play raises issues of the uses of authority, the "hypocrisy of standards," the survival of individuality, and the relations in life between self and others.

In its rulings, the Supreme Court has tried to reinforce the importance of a trial, but the proceedings of the courtroom, except in notorious or well-publicized cases, do not absorb the interest of much of the public. In the majority of cases, the court proceeding is not a great public ceremony or a morality play, and so in the usual situation a trial has fallen into disuse. The development of the pretrial conference in civil cases (actually a trial in chambers) and plea bargaining in criminal cases are indicative of the decline of the public-trial process. In so-called minor offenses the offender frequently pays a fine through the mail, giving rise to the barb that the court is nothing more than a revenue court. In cases when a trial does occur, the courtroom is usually empty, although spectators are occasionally drawn from clearly definable segments of the population.

In modern times, the use of the theater itself as a forum for public, moral judgment has declined in importance and has become rather a place in which private quarrels and agonies are staged. The verdict which events render upon characters in most modern plays often has no relevance beyond the play itself. The function of the old morality play is now essentially presented in other forms. In some fine arts, the central purpose is to instruct or tell the truth. Poet Josef Brodsky, emigré from the Soviet Union, points out that in Russia the church, the system of justice, and several other social institutions have always been in extremely unsatisfactory condition and have not managed to discharge their duties. It happened, he says, that literature was forced to assume many of these functions. "Literature took upon itself the 'instructive' role," he writes. "It became the focus of a people's spiritual life, the arbiter of its moral character."[11]

In sports, wrestling has been a popular substitute of the morality play. To illustrate, a beer drinker, who was recently observed watching a wrestling match on television, slammed his fist on the bar and shouted, "I don't give a damn if it is a fake! Kill the S.O.B." Although he seemed aware that the match was staged, the fan was caught up in the heat of the performance—in the struggle between beauty and ugliness, between good and evil. He was crying for blood, or more mildly, to see justice done.[12]

The role of the criminal trial as morality play was emphasized by the late Philip Q. Roche, a psychiatrist who was also a lifelong student of criminal law. He wrote:

The criminal trial is an operation having a religious meaning essential as a public exercise in which the prevailing moral ideals are dramatized and reaffirmed. The religious meaning is the adjusting of tensional moral conflict within the law-abiding. The conflict is materialized in the actions of the criminal and dissipated in the ritual of guilt fastening, condemnation, and punishment. The ritual is the homologue of the child-parent interaction containing the same motivational mechanisms and rationalizations. In this view, the criminal trial has the function of public edification rather than that of welfare of the individual wrong-doers who pass over its stage in an endless process. In fixed formula and procedure, the trial reiterates the moral parables of our child-rearing and, in the person of the judge, brings to the transgressor a power and punitive enforcement once exercised by the parent. Both judge and parent act as agents of an order defined by the prevailing ethical system.[13]

By and large, the press, television, and radio now function as our public forums, although the court remains to some extent a public forum, and a trial takes the form of a debate of a public issue. Notable examples, past and present, include Oscar Wilde and the issue of homosexuality; Aaron Burr and the power of the Presidency; Scopes and evolution; the Soviet trials of the thirties and party loyalty; the Nuremberg trials and war morality; Eichmann and genocide; Brother Daniel and Jewish identity; Lieutenant Calley and the inhumanity of My Lai; Daniel Ellsberg and Anthony Russo and government control over information. In the United States, the court has also moved into such general areas as desegregation, reapportionment, and the right to medical treatment, assuming the task neglected by other institutions. While the usual run-of-the-mill court trial, like the theater itself, no longer serves as a morality play, the constitutional right to a fair trial and due process continues to serve as a kind of tranquilizer.

Seething passions are unleashed by a wrong, be it real or fancied, and some means are needed to channel and control them. The law, of course, is one of the major institutions designed by man to control his impulses. There is a compelling need for the imposition of punishment, either when there is a strong reason to believe that the behavior in question can be deterred or when noncompliance with a particular norm is generally felt to be so serious that doing nothing will be unacceptable to individuals or groups in the society. To illustrate, murder is considered to be one of the crimes least capable of being deterred, since it is more impulsive than planned, but members of society would not likely tolerate nothing being done about it. Mario Puzo's popular novel, *The Godfather*, opens with Amerigo Bonasera looking to the law, losing faith in it, and then going on his knees to Don Corleone for justice.[14]

Seeking a definition of "justice" brings to mind a colloquy between an examiner and a law-school graduate seeking admission to the bar. To the question, "What is justice?", the applicant said, after a bit of pondering, "I once knew, but now I've forgotten." "What a great loss for jurisprudence!" bemoaned the examiner. "The first person to know, and he's forgotten!" Recognizing Socrates' contribution, the late Mark Van Doren noted that the word *ius* in Latin meant *justice* and *juice*, two apparently unrelated things, and he suggested that they are related in that they both provide a good taste.

In early childhood we complain that things are unfair, and from the way that mother resolves the complaint our concepts of justice begin to formulate. Later on, the guarantee of a fair trial assures us that we will receive fair treatment. Man seems impelled to expect justice, despite, or perhaps out of, his continuing experience of injustice. John F. Kennedy, assassinated at the peak of his life, at one time had said, "All of life is unfair." Jesus was crucified yet he lived the holy life. We all suffer "the slings and arrows of outrageous fortune," but we have, echoing Job, a deep expectation that someone should appoint us a time to secure justice.

At various times and places, the manner of resolution of disputes has differed widely. The development of the judicial process reflects the on-togeny of a ritual, which is, in Erik Erikson's words, "based on sanctified agreement rather than on passing outrage or personal revenge." The ear-lier modes of trial—by ordeal or battle—could be described as then so-cially acceptable but purely ritualistic procedures for preserving the peace by terminating disputes. They could be regarded as methods of determining the truth only on the theory that divine interpretation and intervention brought about the success of the party whose cause was right. But in common estimation the current mode of trial involves, like science, a search for objective truth.

Procedures in early history were entirely formulary, not evidentiary. The oath at one time was the primary mode of proof, its value varying according to a man's rank in society; thus, the oath of a thegn was equal to the oaths of six ceorls. The individual disqualified from taking the oath was put through one of the forms of ordeal, which was an appeal to God to show where the guilt lay. Quite likely, in the Anglo-Saxon age, there were few guilty men who would refuse to confess their guilt when the alternative appeared to be a direct challenge to God. The stress now is on evidentiary substance, but it is tied in with the old stress on evi-dentiary procedure.

To the extent that the court does not have all the relevant evidence, its decision, which nonetheless may be a proper one, will be based on a distorted or lopsided presentation of the case, and it would not even give the appearance of having administered justice fairly. In a political sense, every man is said to have a right to his opinion, but in a court of law neither judge nor jury theoretically have the right to form an opinion in favor of the party having the burden of proof unless he has met this bur-den with good evidence. Only the appellate court judge is obliged to set out reasons for his decision.

Evidence is now called the basis for justice. Professor Oliver Schroe-der, upon his inauguration as 14th President of the American Academy of Forensic Sciences, said that "the greatest challenge of the 1970s is the creation of a system of civil and criminal justice which acquires truthful facts, applies equitable rules of conduct, and decides human contro-versies with just verdicts based on fair and impartial procedures."

NOTES

Note for nonlawyer readers: The reports of cases, scarcely read by the general public, have a technical and uninteresting look about them, but each is a tale of a human tragedy, strange or commonplace. The decisions of the court are called *opinions*; each is a statement by the court of the facts and its ruling, with reasons. The case is recorded under the names of the plaintiff and the defendant, however humble or illustrious they may be. A person sometimes gains immortality from the novelty of the circumstances or the novelty of principle on which the claim was decided. The decisions of the court are published in books called *reports* or *reporters*, and are cited in this manner: *Pavlicic v. Vogtsberger*, 390 Pa. 502, 136 A.2d 127 (1957). Pavlicic and Vogtsberger are the names of the parties involved in the litigation. The intervening *v.* stands for *versus*. The initial number refers to the volume and the latter number to the page in the reporter, followed within parentheses by the year in which the decision was rendered. 2d indicates that the reporter is in a second series. Thus, in the example, the case appears in volume 390 at page 502 of the state reporter (Pennsylvania) and also in volume 136 at page 127 of the second series of the Atlantic regional reports. In this book, case reports and legislation only are cited according to the *Uniform System of Legal Citation*. Cambridge: *Harvard Law Review*, 1967. A reference on legal sources is Roalfe, W. R. (Ed.). *How to Find the Law*. St. Paul, Minn.: West, 1965. The court does not entertain moot or theoretical issues. A party must have standing to bring an action; that is, he must allege such "a personal stake in the outcome of the controversy as to assure that concrete adverseness which sharpens the presentation of issues upon which the court so largely depends for illumination of difficult questions." *Baker v. Carr*, 369 U.S. 186 (1962).

1. Who has not played WAHM (Why Does This Always Happen to Me), or SWYMD (See What You Made Me Do), and its counterpart UGMIT (You Got Me Into This), a game played to perfection by Laurel and Hardy. Marital games include "Harried" (popular with housewives), "Look How Hard I've Tried" (popular with husbands), and "If It Weren't for You" (popular with both spouses)? See Berne, E. *Games People Play*. See also Chapman, A. H. *Put-Offs and Come-Ons*.
2. Arnold, T. The Criminal Trial as a Symbol of Public Morality. In Howard, A. E. (Ed.). *Criminal Justice in Our Time*. P. 39.
3. Sir Edward A. Parry some years ago wrote:
   From the earliest dawn of civilization we find that justice has seen fit to cast her manifestations in a dramatic form. Even today when we think of a trial or a lawsuit we picture it to ourselves in terms of drama, applauding the hero or heroine, execrating the villain of the piece. . . . And as we read the report of a law case we recall the familiar scenery of a court house, the traditional costumes of the characters, and that dramatic setting which we inwardly approve of as essential to the administration of justice.
   Parry, E. A. *The Drama of the Law*. See also Morton, J. D. The Function of Criminal Law in 1962. Canadian Broadcasting Co. lecture, 1962.
4. Smith, M. Attorney Percy Foreman Wins Another Big Case. *Life*, April 1, 1966, p. 92. "The 'art' of the advocate," says Cyril Harvey in his book, *The Advocate's Devil*, "might be defined as 'the art of misleading an audience without actually telling lies.' " There is a saying among lawyers that if the law is against you, pound the evidence; if the evidence is against you, pound the law; if both are against you, pound the table.
5. Seigenthaler, J. *A Search for Justice*. P. 202. In a passage in Henry Cecil's novel, *Friends at Court*, a client thanks his attorney for his help. "But what a lot of time and money," he said, "it has cost to arrive at the truth." "The truth?" said the attorney. "No one said anything about arriving at the truth." The late Professor Edmund M. Morgan of the Harvard Law School used to say that truth is only an ingredient of justice, which is something larger than

truth and far more difficult to attain. See Slovenko, R. The Opinion Rule and Wittgenstein's Tractatus. *U. Miami L. Rev.* 14:1, 1959; revised version in *ETC.* 24:289, 1967.

6. Epstein, J.   Truth in the Courtroom. *Commentary,* Aug. 1969, p. 50. The public has a right to demand only fairness in the procedure, and when a party has had the opportunity of a day in court, the community thenceforth in good conscience can ignore his complaint. The judicial process is a way of resolving conflicting claims that would otherwise disrupt society by self-help or private feud. The process, acceptable to the community, is called justice. Steinberg, H. B. Book Review. *Harv. L. Rev.* 80:477, 1966.

7. Aubert, V.   The Stucture of Legal Thinking. In *Legal Essays, Festschrift Til Frede Castberg,* 1963; Cowan, T.   Jurisprudence in the Teaching of Torts. *J. Legal Ed.* 9:444, 455, 1957.

8. Cowan, T.   Jurisprudence in the Teaching of Torts. *J. Legal Ed.* 9:444, 455, 1957.

9. Wigmore, J.   *A Student's Textbook of the Law of Evidence.* Pp. 10–11. Collingwood puts it thus:
   The methods of criminal detection are not at every point identical with those of scientific history, because their ultimate purpose is not the same. A criminal court has in its hands the life and liberty of a citizen, and in a country where the citizen is regarded as having rights the court is therefore bound to do something and do it quickly. The time taken to arrive at a decision is a factor in the value (that is, the justice) of the decision itself. If any juror says: "I feel certain that a year hence, when we have all reflected on the evidence at leisure, we shall be in a better position to see what it means," the reply will be: "There is something in what you say; but what you propose is impossible. Your business is not just to give a verdict; it is to give a verdict now; and here you stay until you do it." This is why a jury has to content itself with something less than scientific (historical) proof, namely with that degree of assurance or belief which would satisfy it in any of the practical affairs of daily life. Collingwood, R. G.   *The Idea of History.* P. 268.
      The difficulty of determining the proper time for making a decision is illustrated by the administrative regulation of color television. The FCC waited several years for the development of a color system compatible with the black-and-white system. Finally, the FCC felt it could wait no longer and authorized the CBS noncompatible system. RCA's compatible system, economically and scientifically more desirable was still in an experimental stage. RCA attacked the order. The Supreme Court ruled that the FCC had not acted capriciously. [*RCA v. United States,* 341 U.S. 412 (1951).] The CBS system, however, never got off the ground commercially, and the FCC, realizing that it had acted in haste, reversed itself in 1953 and authorized the RCA system.

10. In this case the husband, a scientist, had kept a diary of his dreams for nearly six years, and during this time had recorded the details of nearly one thousand dreams. This diary was confiscated by his wife who proceeded to check carefully the dreams for material which she thought might be incriminating if presented in court. She found a few dreams in which the husband had incestuous relations with some of their young daughters. The wife contended that those dreams proved her husband was an unfit and immoral father who would try to turn his incestuous dreams into reality if allowed future visits with the daughters. She therefore insisted that her husband be denied any form of visitation rights. The psychiatrist on behalf of the husband testified that while there were seven dreams involving incest, approximately 130 involved sexual relationships with adult females, and since this was nearly twenty times the number of incestuous dreams, it seemed as if the dreamer's main sexual interests were clearly of an adult heterosexual type. The judge ruled that the dream diary did not constitute sufficient evidence to deny visitation rights. Van de Castle, R. L.   Sexual Dreams. *Sexual Behavior,* July 1971, p. 14. Among documentation of the importance of dreams in understanding personality development is Bell, A. P., and

Hall, C. S. *The Personality of a Child Molester: An Analysis of Dreams*. Chicago: Aldine-Atherton, 1971. In Shakespeare's *Othello*, Act III, Sc. iii, Iago says, "In sleep I heard him (Cassio) say 'Sweet Desdemona, Let us be wary, let us hide our loves.' " Would this "testimony" of Iago be admissible against Cassio, or Desdemona? The question was presented on a state bar examination. A party's extrajudicial admissions are not conclusive against him, and may be explained, limited, qualified and contradicted; a party may always explain the circumstances under which inconsistent statements or claims were made and reconcile them with his testimony. *Aide v. Taylor*, 7 N.W.2d 757 (Minn. 1943).

In the witch trials of the 17th century, an accuser's hallucinations, dreams and mere fancies would be accepted in court as factual proof not of the psychological condition of the accuser but of the behavior of the accused. There was no disproof against this sort of "proof." If an accuser says, "Your shape came to my room last night," the accused had no defense. No conceivable alibi can be furnished for the whereabouts of a shape, one's airy substance. Starkey, M. L. *The Devil in Massachusetts*. New York: Knopf, 1949. P. 54. See also de Becker, R. *The Understanding of Dreams and Their Influence on the History of Man*. New York: Bell, 1958.

11. *New York Times Magazine*, Oct. 1, 1972, p. 11.
12. Stone, G. P., and Oldenberg, R. A. Wrestling. In Slovenko, R., and Knight, J. A. (Eds.). *Motivations in Play, Games and Sports*. Pp. 503–532.
13. Roche, P. O. *The Criminal Mind*. P. 245.
14. Report on Crime and Punishment in America Prepared for the American Friends Service Committee, *Struggle for Justice*. Dr. Karl Menninger contends that as much as penalties are needed for deterrents and public protection, and even for a part of the morality-play effect, whenever the penalty is too great and produces a backlash of bitterness and retaliation, it does far more harm than good in several directions. See Menninger, K. A. *The Crime of Punishment*.

2. Psychiatric Expert Testimony and the Adversary System

EVERY person owes the duty of aiding in the settlement of controversies; it is an important public function. The law gives to the tribunal, and to the attorney as its officer, the power to summon anyone (except the President) and to compel him to answer, as a rule, any question. The only specific constitutional exception to a witness testifying before a grand jury or at a trial is the privilege not to give evidence against oneself. Another exception, although not based on any constitutional mandate, is the privilege given a witness to keep secret certain information acquired in some confidential relationships.

Distinguishing Anglo-American common-law justice is the importance attached to the function of a public trial, the right to confront witnesses, and the use of formal rules of evidence. Continental legal procedure, both of the noncommunist and communist worlds, is without the kind of formalism found in the common-law system. Objections such as "inadmissible evidence," "hearsay," "opinion," or "leading question," customary in an Anglo-American trial, are unknown. In the view of Anglo-American law, the key to a fair trial is the presentation of evidence according to formal rules of evidence, the opportunity to use cross-examination, rebuttal evidence, and argument to meet adverse materials. The confrontation clause of the Sixth Amendment prescribes a cross-examining procedure, which is the very heart of the adversary system.

This adversary proceeding, in an impartial forum, provides a mechanism by which differences can be settled in a decision-making process that people generally trust. It provides a means of making even big government and big business accountable. It buttresses the individual's self-image, his sense of worth, by being able to assert a legal right in a proceeding where he has reasonable equality with that of the opponent. It is the modern-day scene where David may defeat Goliath. To be sure, there are critics, particularly among losers. Charlie Chaplin in his autobiography said of the paternity suit that went against him, "Listening to the legal abracadabra of both attorneys, it seemed to me a game they were playing and that I had little to do with it." Ralph Ginzburg said, after having served eight months of a three-year sentence for sending obscene materials through the mail, "Justice in this country is not a beautiful, blindfolded woman but a deaf, blind old man."

Under the adversary system the judge acts as arbiter to assure conformity to those rules of fair play that have evolved over the centuries. The jury then decides the issues on the basis of those facts which the judge permits them to hear. Simply put, the adversary system is a process of contention in which the role of the lawyer is to initiate suit following the dispute, raise the issues, and propel the controversy. In this system, the judge does not venture forth like a Don Quixote seeking justice as he does under the inquisitorial system which prevails in most countries. The inquisitorial judge has the responsibility to "arrive at the truth by his own exertions in conjunction with those of the official prosecutor," well illustrated in the Brigitte Bardot movie *La Verité*; but the judge in the adversary system decides the issues when and as the lawyers present them. Experimental studies lend support to the claim that an adversary form of presentation, in contradistinction to an inquisitorial presentation, counteracts bias in decisionmakers.

The physical setting reflects the system. Under the adversary system, in civil and criminal cases, the chairs of the parties in the courtroom are situated on the same level, without benefit of elevation above the floor, and are equidistant from the judge. The parallel location of the parties is designed to indicate to judge and jury that the word of one counsel—prosecutor (plaintiff in civil cases) or defense counsel—carries no more weight than that of the other. The scales of justice are thus held evenly. In other countries, operating under the inquisitorial system, the prosecutor has a place well above that of the counsel for defense, and he carries by virtue of his location a certain majesty, hardly distinguishable from that of the judge. A judge sits elevated, a position communicating dominance or superiority, because his symbolic authority and judgment under law is final. Men of superior rank have been addressed as "Your *High*ness."

In the Anglo-American courtroom arena, the rules governing the action are as formal and ritualistic as those of a tournament or a game of chess. Each side is charged with presenting the strongest possible case on its own behalf and expects to be countered with the strongest possible case by the adversary, so that conditions like those of the ancient tournament are created. The adversary proceeding requires that the lawyer-gladiators, in carrying out their task, be fair or sporting.

The adversary system is based on the theory that truth (or viewpoints) attainable in a courtroom emerges best out of the open combat of ideas. While physicians are trained to discover medical truth, lawyers are trained in representing any point of view. The theory of the adversary system, as Professor Edmund Morgan once put it, is that "each litigant is most interested and will be most effective in seeking, discovering, and presenting the materials which will reveal the strength of his own case and the weakness of his adversary's case, so that the truth will emerge to the impartial tribunal that makes the decision." In another oft-quoted observation, the late Judge Jerome Frank commented:

> The best way for a court to discover the facts in a suit is to have each side strive as hard as it can, in a keenly partisan spirit, to bring to the court's attention the evidence favorable to that side. . . . The "fight" theory of justice is a sort of legal laissez-faire. . . . Legal laissez-faire theory assumes that government can safely rely on the "individual enterprise" of individual litigants to insure that court orders will be grounded on all the practical, attainable, relevant facts.

He went on, however, to add:

> Most of us have come to distrust, in the economic field, ultra let-alone-ism, the ultra laissez-faire theory with its antisocial concept of an "economic man." For observation of social realities has shown that the basic postulates of that theory, although in part correct, are inadequate as exclusive postulates. I think that, in like fashion, observation of courtroom realities shows that the postulates of legal laissez-faire are insufficient as exclusive postulates. We should retain what there is of value in the fighting theory of justice, eliminating what is socially harmful. . . . [T]he fight should not so dominate a lawsuit that it leads to the nondiscovery of important evidence and the distortion of testimony.[1]

Summoning a specialist or expert witness against his will, either as partisan expert or amicus curiae, to give his professional opinion on the issues involved, gives rise to the pragmatic question whether or not he may refuse to testify unless a reasonable fee be paid, beyond the ordinary witness fee. He may contend that by coming to court to testify he has lost office time and income, which the ordinary witness fee would not approach, and that this results in an unconstitutional taking of property. However, when he makes no special preparation but is called upon only to testify as to what he knows, he is entitled of right only to what is given any ordinary witness. As a practical matter, however, an advocate wants a cooperative expert and that requires payment, sometimes in advance. Money is the best way to please an expert but even that is not easy, for a lot of good experts are already rich.[2]

Securing prepared expert testimony is thus relatively expensive and, as a consequence, is usually unavailable to the indigent, except in personal-injury litigation, when the attorney for the plaintiff covers the expense in the belief that he has a good case. In criminal cases, a number of Supreme Court decisions emphasizing the rights of the accused are making trial judges more cautious about rejecting a defense request for psychiatric examination. The fact remains, however, that to the extent that experts affect the outcome, the indigent is at a disadvantage.

The potential use of expert testimony expands as man gains wider knowledge of his world and as the world becomes more complicated. In *Bananas*, Woody Allen is a products-tester trying out electrically heated toilet seats and coffins with piped-in music. The modern age being a bit much for all of us, it is not surprising that modern litigation requires more expert opinion evidence than ever before, whatever the type of case. Not only is reliance on expert witnesses increasing, but also new types of experts are developing. The method by which experts are utilized is generating controversy, however. Before trial by jury was much developed, there seem to have been two modes of using the expert knowledge that did exist: first, to select as jurymen such persons as were especially fitted by experience to know the class of facts which were before them; and second, to call to the aid of the court skilled persons whose opinions it might adopt or not as it pleased. The existence of the judge's power to call witnesses generally included the power to call expert witnesses who were regarded originally as amici curiae (friends of the court). Centuries ago the English courts called on physicians to help determine whether a defendant was bewitched.

PARTICIPATION IN TEST CASE OR AS AMICUS CURIAE

The use of partisan experts called by the adversary parties has resulted in the controversial "battle of the experts," alienating many professionals from the judicial process. The role of the professional as expert in a test case, however, or as amicus curiae is not to be neglected. In addition to testifying, professionals in the pertinent field can offer invaluable suggestions to an attorney preparing an amicus curiae brief on a point of law or of fact for the information of the judge. In recent decades, the role of the amicus curiae brief has been expanded, and indeed, it is quite common now to see organizational presentation of a brief. Under this modified adversary system, the brief, as a form of information gathering, is the judicial counterpart of lobbying and congressional hearing in the legislative process. Fairly speaking, it is often a "political statement" or "lobbying before the court."[3]

Permission to participate as a friend of the court is and has always been a matter of grace rather than of right. The theory of trial by duel between two contestants precludes an unlimited right of third persons to intervene or file a brief. "The fundamental principle underlying legal procedure," one court observed, "is that parties to a controversy shall have the right to litigate the same, free from the interference of strangers." Chief Justice Burger and many other judges tend to feel that the role of the court is not to decide broad social issues—rather it is to decide a contest between two litigants—and they want "friends" to remain outside the courtroom.

Access to the judicial process on the part of third-party individuals or organizations is an extension of the view that the law is a process of social choice and policy making. The outcome of litigation indirectly affects interests other than those formally represented. Groups organized to promote altruistic goals are likely, as amici, to represent important widespread public interests. Organizational participation in the judicial process focuses attention on the judge's decision, and as a consequence, he is particularly cautious and deliberate in these cases. The National Association for the Advancement of Colored People, almost from its inception, has participated as amicus curiae in litigation. The American Civil Liberties Union early found the amicus curiae brief a useful instrument in drawing widespread attention to its cause. The American Jewish Congress over the past years has been among the most active filers of amicus curiae briefs. Organizational activity in the legal process finds a broad new field with the recent development of the class action, which allows representation of everyone in a similar position.

Moreover, while the party, and not the court, is responsible under the adversary system for gathering and presenting facts, there are many facts which need to be supplemented or cannot be established by formal proof. The doctrine of judicial notice recognizes the right or the necessity of the judge to notice evidence outside the record which is "a matter of general knowledge." The judicial notice apparatus, however, does not work well unless it is fed with information. Judge Frank of the Second Circuit once observed that judicial notice often amounts to nothing more than "cocktail-hour knowledge." He suggested that "competently to inform ourselves, we should have a staff of investigators like those supplied to administrative agencies."

Almost any case can be used to illustrate the need for, and the propriety of, supplying the court with information. The usual method of establishing adjudicative facts, the facts of the particular case, is through the introduction of evidence, ordinarily consisting of the testimony of witnesses, whereas judicial notice is the usual method in the courtroom of finding legislative facts, which are those facts having relevance to legal reasoning and the lawmaking process, whether in the formulation of a legal principle, or ruling by a judge or court, or in the enactment of a legislative body. In judicial lawmaking a prominent illustration of taking notice of a legislative fact is *Durham v. United States,* a decision subsequently cast aside, where Judge Bazelon, without support in the evidence developed at the trial, declared: "Medico-legal writers in large numbers . . . present convincing evidence that the right-and-wrong test is 'based on an entirely obsolete and misleading conception of the nature of insanity.'" The court had no hesitation in using this "convincing evidence" even though it was not in the record. In the landmark case of *Wolf v. Colorado,* Supreme Court Justice Murphy wrote to district attorneys of various cities to learn of police practices there and obtained from their replies information which he used to deal with the issue of illegally obtained evidence at trial. In the case of *Roth v. United States,* decided in 1957, when the Court first dealt directly with the issue of obscenity, it reasoned that "implicit in the history of the First Amendment is the rejection of obscenity as utterly without redeeming social importance." In the historic case in 1954 of *Brown v. Board of Education of Topeka,* the Court cited Kenneth B. Clark and Gunnar Myrdal on the adverse effect of school racial segregation on personality development. Sociological and psychological theories also controlled the Court's separate-but-equal decision in *Plessy v. Ferguson,* decided in 1896, even though these theories were neither formally presented to the Court nor given formal recognition.

The American Medical Association, American Psychiatric Association, American Psychological Association, and American Orthopsychiatric Association (Ortho) at one time or another have entered as amici on various mental-health issues. These associations, however, have no rational scheme for submitting amici briefs or instituting suit but do so when attention is called by their attorneys, staffs, or interested members to a particular case judged directly relevant to its field, and if there is sufficient time and money. One or another of these associations—in a happenstance, often fortuitous manner—has submitted briefs on issues of criminal responsibility, competency to stand trial, admissibility of expert testimony by psychologists, psychological test validity in assessing employment placement, privileged confidential communication, services to the mentally retarded, adequacy of treatment in mental hospitals and mental-retardation institutions, peonage in mental institutions, psycho-surgery, capital punishment, unusual punishment in solitary confine-ment, denial of admission of candidate to medical school because of a prior mental-hospital stay, imprisonment for possession of marijuana, and abortion. In addition, these associations on occasion have offered sundry proposals for model legislation.

The Supreme Court's 1972 rulings on competency to stand trial in *Jackson v. Indiana* and the death penalty in *Furman v. Georgia* (which we later discuss), draw heavily on the issues formulated and researched in the amicus briefs. In fact, most of the issues discussed by the Court in *Jackson v. Indiana* were not touched on by attorneys for the state or for the defendant but were raised only in Ortho's amicus brief. The brief called the Court's attention to the broad implications of the procedure used in commitment for incompetency to stand trial, and the Court, al-though it did not permit filing of the brief, responded by addressing it-self to these issues.

While it may encumber the judicial process, many courts are grateful for the participation of amicus curiae. A court's opinion often incorpo-rates verbatim the amicus brief, which has come, in the style of the Brandeis brief, to represent the intersection of scholarship and advocacy. An amicus may enter at the trial or appellate level although rarely is af-forded the opportunity to participate on the trial level, as it did in *Wyatt v. Stickney*, the right-to-treatment case, where it was actively engaged in the proceeding and presented numerous witnesses on all aspects of the case. In helping to formulate minimum medical and constitutional standards in hospital treatment, the court expressed gratitude for ex-emplary service to Ortho, ACLU, American Psychological Association, and American Association on Mental Deficiency.

Today, individuals look to their organizations to represent and further their professional interests and concerns. As individuals, they have neither the time nor the inclination to pursue a matter that does not directly and immediately affect their pocketbooks and they have come to expect organizational representation in the courts on general profes-sional matters. While there has been much criticism of the role of men-tal-health professionals as expert witnesses in the adversary process, it is at the same time recognized that in some way their viewpoint should enter the judicial process.

Under the regulations [§1.501(c)(3)] of the Internal Revenue Ser-vice, the status of contributions as gifts and the charitable classification of an association would not be jeopardized by involvement in court proceed-ings, either on its own behalf or as amicus curiae. There are, though, other limitations placed upon an organization as a nonprofit, tax-exempt organization which should be noted. It may not use any "substantial portion of its resources" in attempting to influence the legislative process. It may produce educational and informational materials, but it may not lead crusades or propaganda campaigns. It may respond to requests to testify before legislative hearings, and members of the staff may voluntarily appear, but only as individuals and not representing the organization. If these restrictions are too confining, an organization could establish a coordinate activity organization, which would not be tax-exempt, and thus could become involved in political, propaganda, or legislative campaigns. Thus the ACLU and the NAACP are, respectively, the activist organizations of the ACLU Foundation and the NAACP Legal Defense Fund.

Ortho is currently carrying out a part of its role in the developing use of legal approaches to critical mental-health issues as a sponsor of the National Council on the Rights of the Mentally Impaired along with the ACLU Foundation and the Center for Law and Social Policy. The Council (now called Mental Health Law Project), established in early 1972, is developing test cases in the courts, educating lawyers for practice in the mental-health field, centralizing information for lawyers in the field, and developing models for legal activity. At the same time, Ortho is focusing on the education of the mental-health professional as to the issues in which law can be used as an instrument of mental-health policy development.

As an avenue of publicity, amici briefs are often published in the *Congressional Record*—any congressman can put anything in the *Record*, and on request he will usually do so. The *Record* makes it possible to publish at a low printing price (the cost absorbed by the public). Each day, within thirteen hours of the close of debate, congressional presses turn out 49,000 copies of another thick edition of the *Record*. While production may be impressive, content unfortunately is not. In effect, the *Record* is a subsidiary xeroxing service for congressmen, producing by the thousands whatever item they choose. Nader's Study Group, which calls the *Record* a big charade, says that shrewd doctors soon will learn to stock their waiting rooms with copies of the *Record*. In any event, the *Record* is a means to heighten visibility and citizen consciousness of an issue, which is also the goal of much litigation.

PARTICIPATION AS PARTISAN EXPERT

While the amicus role is developing, partisan experts called by the contesting parties remain the familiar source of expert testimony. Under the adversary system, if one's expert takes an impartial or middle position, and the other side goes to its extreme, then where is one, except up the proverbial creek?

In a battle, it is necessary to take account of the adversary. An expert who takes a neutral role does his party a disservice, for the opposing party's expert will undoubtedly assume his role as advocate and his advocacy would go without challenge. Hence, when a witness chooses to testify as an expert for a party, he is expected to do so under the terms of the adversary system or he should not participate. It is only in recognizing his role as partisan advocate that an expert can testify responsibly in the courtroom.

The role of the expert may be to reconstruct the past, analyze the present, or predict the future. In doing this, he may offer testimony of two general kinds: testimony as to facts and opinion testimony. The admissibility of each rests upon different theories. Expert testimony as to facts is admissible because special skill and experience are needed for the understanding of certain matters. For example, any person of ordinary understanding can testify as to whether a man had a cut or to the color of stains that may have appeared on his clothes. It requires special experience and knowledge, however, to say what arteries, nerves, or bones were injured and to determine whether the stains, if yellow, were due to urine or semen, or if brown, were human blood. Because the ordinary witness is not capable of understanding the particular matter, the expert is needed, but his special knowledge must be shown before he is permitted to testify as an expert.

As a general rule of evidence, opinion testimony is inadmissible. The ordinary witness presents the facts, and the judge or jury is to draw the inferences or conclusions from such facts. A parallel may be seen in the doctor-patient relationship, as when a doctor may say to a patient, "I'll do the diagnosing, if you don't mind. Just tell me what ails you." In many instances, however, it is not possible for the court to form an intelligent judgment because of the difficulty of the question involved, and the opinion of those skilled in that particular subject may be obtained for assistance. For example, the jury would be incapable of determining whether or not death resulted from a particular cut, even though it had before it a description of the wound; hence the opinion of a medical person is of assistance to the jury. Here the function of opinion testimony is advising the jury rather than proving facts.

The problem of expert testimony, particularly that of a psychiatric character, whether as to facts or opinion, is somewhat different in criminal than in civil cases because of certain constitutional privileges of the accused. On account of the defendant's privilege against self-incrimination, the expert witness for the state in a criminal prosecution is much more restricted when the defendant's mental, rather than physical, condition is in issue. The accused may be compelled to submit to a physical examination by the medical witness for the prosecution since this does not involve testimonial compulsion.[4] The accused cannot be compelled to answer any questions asked by the expert in a mental examination, however, because this would violate his privilege against self-incrimination.[5] If the defendant wishes to plead insanity, he must submit to a psychiatric examination; but the psychiatrist may testify only on the issue of mental status and may not reveal any statement made to him as to the commission of the offense.

Currently, the bulk of civil proceedings involves personal injury litigation, with domestic relations a distant second. In personal injury litigation and in workmen's compensation cases, the physician for various reasons is generally reluctant about serving as an expert witness. He dislikes taking time from his practice. He is reluctant to oppose openly another physician's testimony, and he resents the confrontation implicit in cross-examination. He is, moreover, annoyed at having to answer "Yes" or "No" in a dogmatic way. He is king of the roost in the hospital. The doctor in the hospital goes on GRAND ROUNDS (capitalized on notices), and he is unaccustomed to being badgered or humiliated. He is so conscious of status that he is even offended if he is addressed as "Mister" instead of "Doctor." As a result only a small percentage of physicians represent the entire profession in court, although in recent years a number of organizations have sprung up around the country that make available a coterie of expert witnesses. They are sometimes known as the "old horses" of the courtroom, representing regularly either plaintiffs or defendants. They are diagnosed by their colleagues as "frustrated lawyers."

In criminal proceedings, the psychiatrist is the principal expert witness who is summoned, but he may be reluctant (as are most lawyers) to have contact with the criminal element. The psychologist tends to be more interested in participating, but although qualified to serve as an expert witness, he is often challenged on his competency. The practice of psychiatry, like medicine generally, is a booming business, and the psychiatrist has no inclination to become involved with indigent or dangerous people; he is like everyman concerned about his image. Also as noted, there is the fear of humiliation at the hands of the lawyers, and there is the uncertainty about the psychological nature of crime or the relevance of actual evidence and past crime. As a witness, the psychiatrist is often identified in the mind of the public as someone hired to cheat justice by testifying that the defendant is not guilty by reason of insanity. In addition, the criminal offender usually tends to be uneducated, simple, nonverbal, uninteresting, and as a consequence, does not appeal to psychiatry, which is a profession essentially based on talking.

CRITICISM OF PSYCHIATRIST IN ADVERSARY ROLE

Criticism of the role of the psychiatrist in the courtroom, which comes from both within and without the psychiatric profession, is of a special nature. Fyodor Dostoevsky, in *The Brothers Karamazov*, wrote that there was an element of comedy in having a psychiatrist in the courtroom. It is frequently argued that the giving of testimony to affect the verdict is the least helpful and least productive of the tasks that could evolve for the psychiatrist, and that if he is to participate in the trial process, it should be either in the pretrial or postverdict phases, at which time consultation might be made on disposition and implementation.

Among others, Dr. Karl Menninger suggests that psychiatrists be excluded entirely from the courtroom, not just because psychiatrists do not like to be disputed by colleagues, badgered and discredited on cross-examination by attorneys, or suspected of being purchasable, but also because questions relating to guilt, competence, and responsibility are moral or legal questions, not medical or psychiatric ones. While at one time expressing great optimism about the possibilities of the Durham decision (discussed in chapter 5), in opening up psychiatric testimony on criminal responsibility, Menninger since then has urged psychiatrists to keep out of the courtroom. "I think with a little skillful business management," he said, "I might run my worldly possessions up to the half million mark if I would agree to testify in all the cases that want me. But I don't believe in it, and I won't do it, and that's just too bad for my pocketbook. . . . [T]hese court hearings put psychologists and psychiatrists at a great disadvantage. It's not our way of looking at things. It's not our way of talking. I don't want to dispute a colleague in front of a lot of people, but I would love to discuss the case with him in private."[6]

In *The Crime of Punishment*, Menninger wrote:

We [psychiatrists] don't belong [in the courtroom]. We cannot function effectively there. It is not our proper sphere of action. We do not understand the language addressed to us nor convey what we intend to and think we do, using the language we employ. Our performance in the courtroom ritual is a continuation of what is really a fraudulent, discriminatory, undemocratic procedure—that of trying to manipulate psychiatric categories and legal sanctions for the special benefit of selected individuals.

There is a law-psychiatry division at the Menninger Foundation, but "psychiatrists have no business appearing in court, at least not at trials," Menninger has asserted. While urging the court to keep all psychiatrists out of trials, he suggests that doctors and their assistants examine the defendant outside the courtroom and render a report to the court, which will express their view of the offender: his potentialities, his shortcomings, and possible remedies. Menninger has urged:

> If we doctors cannot agree, let us disagree in private and submit majority and minority reports. That probably will not be necessary; our differences are going to be on minor points. We are not going to raise legal issues like "sanity" and "responsibility" because we are not going to talk legal jargon. Nor should we talk [psychiatric] jargon. We should try to say in simple English why we think this man has acted in this way so different from the rest of us, and what we think can be done to change his pattern. [The court] will then decide if we have been persuasive and make possible by order what [it thinks] is the most promising recommendation.[7]

According to Dr. Lawrence Kolb, Director of the New York State Psychiatric Institute, psychiatrists "contribute to the erosion of the force of law" by the "unwitting continuance" of the practice of testifying in court as to a defendant's mental state at the time he allegedly committed a criminal act. It is his position that "the appearance of the psychiatrist on the stand in adversary positions damages the concept of justice under our law" and damages the respect psychiatry "is due as a consequence of the vast increase in our knowledge as regards human behavior, the motivations driving that behavior, and the sources of its social aberrations. It does the public respect for law little good to have a psychiatrist or psychiatrists appearing on the stands to support or deny the plea of insanity as a defense when the defendant is accused of assassination or a series of grisly murders," Kolb continued. "Even worse is the conflicting testimony given in certain cases wherein the suspicion rests that the scientific and professional posture of the specialty has been perverted through the promise of a fee for services rendered." He claims that criticism of psychiatry by judges and lawyers stems from psychiatrists "accepting the role of expert witness to questions largely unanswerable by our special knowledge." He says that growing numbers of young psychiatrists do not wish to "take part in a process which forces them into adversary positions or close to the point of professional perjury."[8]

In this spirit, Dr. William A. Woodruff of the University of Vermont Department of Psychiatry says:

> There is a considerable body of opinion in both the legal and psychiatric professions that the present state of affairs cannot last much longer. The spectacle of so-called experts being caused to reveal their personal idiosyncrasies and the general inadequacies of the psychiatric profession in the glaring light of publicity which the open court permits is disconcerting, to say the least. The practice of prosecutor and defense attorney alike in utilizing particular psychiatrists with particular theoretical approaches to serve their ends is valid enough under the present system but guaranteed to bring the profession as a whole into disrepute. But it should be recognized that those psychiatrists who take part in these proceedings are as much responsible for this state of affairs as the legal system. . . . As Judge Bazelon, author of the Durham rule, has recently pointed out, there is considerable doubt as to the validity of using psychiatrists in their present role. And since there is such a poor level of efficiency in the present system, the need for a revision is overripe.[9]

The Advisory Committee on the *Federal Rules of Evidence* says that "the practice of shopping for experts, the venality of some experts, and the reluctance of many reputable experts to involve themselves in litigation have been matters of deep concern." Though the contention is made that court-appointed experts acquire an aura of infallibility to which they are not entitled, the trend is increasingly to provide for their use. The Massachusetts Briggs Law requires impaneling "impartial experts who will render a scientifically sound and unbiased presentation of the medical facts," thus removing from the courtroom the conflicting views of the prosecution- and defense-retained experts. The Advisory Committee observes that while experience indicates that actual court appointment of an expert is generally a relatively infrequent occurrence, the assumption is made that the availability of the procedure in itself decreases the need for resorting to it. The ever-present possibility that the judge *may* appoint an expert in a given case inevitably exerts a sobering effect on the expert witness of a party and upon the person utilizing his services.[10]

Experience of the law reveals that there is almost no subject which cannot be viewed in at least two ways. Articulate statements in favor of retaining psychiatric testimony within the adversary system have been made by, among others, Dean Abraham Goldstein and forensic psychiatrists Henry Davidson, Bernard Diamond, and Alan A. Stone. Listing the pros and cons of the controversy over the psychiatrist's role in the courtroom indicates powerful arguments on each side, a fact which points up the very virtue of the adversary system.

The adversary system, the battle of the experts which it entails, and the frequent reversals on appeal may all reflect the natural working of the human mind. Reversals on account of "trial error" are not due to any stupidity of the trial judge. Freud has shown that ambivalence is the normal manner of human thought. The "adversary rumination" keeps the law in correspondence with human nature. Erik Erikson observed, "The conflicting evidence which parades past the paternal (or parental) judge, the fraternal jury, and the chorus of the public, matches the unceasing inner rumination with which we watch ourselves."[11]

There are at least two sides to every story; the obsessive-compulsive individual may find even more than two sides. Life is Janus-faced. In every war there have been virtuous and reasonable men earnestly fighting on both sides. Socrates would allow an adversary to pick any side of an argument. In the same spirit, Ralph Waldo Emerson would give a lecture on one side of a subject, then on the other side. The dialectic of thesis and antithesis is the basis of Hegel's philosophy. Don Quixote's practical sidekick, Sancho Panza, knew the ambivalence of taboos. Apparently for every proverb—that pithy summary of popular wisdom—there is another which contradicts it flatly, as for instance, "a rolling stone gathers no moss," as against "the traveling bee gets the honey"; or "look before you leap," as against "he who hesitates is lost"; "The Lord loveth a cheerful giver," but "fools and their money are soon parted"; "absence makes the heart grow fonder," but "out of sight, out of mind."[12]

The psychiatrist who shirks testifying may be failing an individual just at the moment that he is needed most. His testimony may be subject to criticism but, "no witness is expected to hit a home run." Moreover, whether in or out of court, working with the court offers an unparalleled opportunity to study human behavior as litigation of any kind represents a breakdown in social functioning that needs to be understood. Avoiding the courtroom is to close one door, a very important one, on the study of disturbed behavior and on the application of current knowledge to the legal and social institutions. In addition, the courtroom provides an arena to inform the public, to initiate legal reforms, and to influence public attitudes.

ATTACKS ON PSYCHIATRIC TESTIMONY

Several attacks are made on psychiatric testimony. One attack concerns psychiatrists who testify for publicity's sake. Having the public in mind, their testimony may be so skewed as not to be trusted. For another, it is alleged that psychiatric testimony is not understandable to lay juries. It is often called *gobbledygook*. Even the key defense witness in the murder trial of Sirhan Sirhan conceded that the jury might have trouble accepting his testimony that Sirhan killed Senator Kennedy while in a self-induced hypnotic trance. He readily acknowledged that his testimony seemed an "absurd, preposterous story, unlikely and incredible." He was not alone in his confession. Psychiatrists testifying on both sides in the Sirhan trial admitted that their statements must have sounded incredible to the jury.[13]

Another criticism is that a psychiatric prognosis is unreliable. The generally low level of accuracy of prediction is said to be "by now so well known as not to need documentation." The psychiatrist rarely has follow-up knowledge of the results of his evaluations or treatment, and is particularly vulnerable to questioning on his follow-up techniques and the percentage of evaluations which have proved right or wrong by independent objective criteria. Yet a great part of the information sought from a psychiatrist by the court involves prediction. In many areas, particularly those involving the psychiatrist, the legal process seeks a prediction of future events rather than a determination of who did what at some time in the past. In child custody cases, for example, a judgment is based on the "best interests of the child," which looks to the future. In divorce cases based on "breakdown of the marriage," a prediction is made as to the reconcilability of the partners. In criminal-law administration, a prediction is sought of the likelihood that the offender will commit another crime and a judgment as to the seriousness of that potential crime.

It is a common conception that particular psychiatric labels have a predictive value indicating dangerousness. As certain mental disorders are characterized by agitated, threatening, frightened, or impulsive behavior, it is thought that they indicate dangerousness. Thus, in proceedings respecting release of a person who has been committed to a mental hospital after acquittal by reason of insanity, the opinion is expressed, for example, in reasoning that is circular, that the person is "a paranoid schizophrenic," and therefore potentially dangerous.

There are no absolutes in the prediction of human behavior. The psychiatrist or other social scientist is not a computer that can calculate the behavior of trends as they relate to each other, projecting them into the future. Even statistical results tell us nothing about the single instance, and it is the single case with which a trial deals. The human situation is open; all the parameters are neither fixed nor known, hence there is fallibility in prediction. There is little warrant for the belief that there are iron laws of history, or that we know them well enough to allow projections of any great reliability. Most of the turning points of history, great and small, were surprises to both their participants and the analysts of the day. Social scientists marked Detroit as one of the least vulnerable cities to a race riot; two years later the place exploded. No one imagined that Richard M. Nixon would, when President, exchange toasts with Chou En-lai in Peking and sleep at the Kremlin in Moscow.

A typological construction is theoretically supposed to provide several things: a description or diagnosis, an etiological explanation, and a prognosis. In considerable measure, a medical label—e.g., diabetes—does furnish a description, information about etiology, suggested treatment, and prognosis, and it is expected that psychiatric labels should do the same. But no psychiatric label can deal with all these dimensions simultaneously and relate them to one another functionally. Psychiatric typology like criminal typology (e.g., rapist) deals with behavior, and behavior is a complex function of variables at all levels of abstraction—individual, social, and cultural.

It is also claimed that psychiatric testimony is tenuous because of the complexity and vagueness of the data elicited. The only material which impresses some as being at all scientific or objective is the more concrete evidence of the auxiliary aides of psychotherapy, such as neurological examination, chemical analysis, and psychological experiment. To be sure, there is no way to test will power or the inside of a person's mind, as can be done with blood pressure. Nor can psychiatric labels exactly meet the case since people do not group themselves snugly into behavior categories. Hence, there are significant differences in the diagnosis and psychiatric labels that various psychiatrists would apply to the same individual. A recent study found that experienced psychiatrists disagreed in 75 percent of the cases in which they attempted to relate psychiatric categories to present mental condition.[14] Another study claims that "psychiatric diagnosis at present is so unreliable as to merit very serious question when classifying, studying, and treating patients' behavior and outcomes."[15] This leaves the psychiatrist open to a question calling for an admission that other data may not have been noticed or may not have been remembered when the psychiatrist framed his opinion.

A diagnostic framework suitable for treatment or for research may be quite inappropriate for forensic purposes. Merely because diagnostic categories exist does not mean that they represent objective facts, or that they must be used in law. The degree of diagnostic precision of a test depends on its proper use, and this is often subjective. In forming his opinion, the psychiatrist will often rely on psychological tests (such as Rorschach, MMPI) carried out by another specialist, a psychologist. This opens up questions as to the interpretation of these tests, the role of intuition, the validity of these tests in measuring or assessing a legal issue, the reliability of the employed tests, or psychological tests in general, and the adequacy of such tests in evaluating members of minority groups or subcultures other than those on which the given tests were validated.

TACTICAL USE OF TESTIMONY

Many psychiatrists wonder if their testimony makes any difference anyway in the legal process or if they are simply being used as a ploy. They have respect for the law, which they interpret to mean a literal reading of the law; hence they question any tactical use in law of the concept of mental illness, whatever may be the nonlaw tactical uses.

Persons labeled *schizophrenic* are known to be concretistic in language and thought ("don't put all your eggs in one basket because they might break"), but curiously psychiatrists seem to take a similar literal-minded approach in interpreting rules of law. It is almost like when one asks another how he is feeling and the question is taken literally when a greeting is simply being extended. Transference phenomena illustrate that things are not as they appear—e.g., Anthony Quinn's psychiatrist initially appeared to him to be a Texas cop. Freudian interpretation is based, Ricoeur has pointed out, on the assumption that the patient intends to hide the truth, but psychiatrists generally seem to feel that the law should never be devious like the unconscious. To develop a sense of trust, child psychiatrists insist that parents be honest with their children; thus, children are to be told that Santa Claus is a real make-believe person, not that he is a real person. The psychiatrist's view of the law may stem from the Freudian ideal calling for honesty in interpersonal relations. Oscar Wilde observed, though, that a person who calls a spade a spade may be fit only to use one.

The law is not a threadbare and singular device outside the boundaries of society, doling out absolute judgments within a rule-enclosed courtroom. Supreme Court Justice Felix Frankfurter in his *Reminiscences* had this to say about sociologists and their view of the legal process: "You damned sociologists, you who want to get it all nice and fine on paper, you haven't learned how much in this world is determined by nonsyllogistic reasoning, or without conscious exploration of a problem with a view to reaching a logical conclusion. You fellows haven't learned that. You think we're just rationalistic—not merely reasonable, but rationalistic—automata of a logical process."

While strong reasons are normally required to override precedential history, courts tend to be result-oriented. An issue of significance could hardly be decided without giving consideration to the consequences which will flow from a decision. Logic, except in a formal sense, decides no case. Logic is a system of thought; it is a means, not an end.

In considerable measure, a judicial opinion is an exercise in rhetoric. Freud pointed out that man is capable of devising good reasons for anything. There is an old admonition, "Watch what we do, not what we say," which applies to the courts as well as to anyone else. Each case is to be examined, not as an entity unto itself, but as a part of a whole where the position in accord with societal notions of reasonableness always seems to triumph. No more fitting comment on this approach could be found than the observation of Supreme Court Justice Oliver Wendell Holmes in his classic, *The Common Law,* in which he says: "The very considerations which judges most rarely mention, and always with an apology, are the secret root from which the law draws all the juices of life. I mean, of course, considerations of what is expedient for the community concerned. Every important principle which is developed by litigation is, in fact and at bottom, the result of more or less definitely understood views of public policy; most generally, to be sure, under our practice and traditions, the unconscious result of instinctive preferences and inarticulate convictions, but none the less traceable to views of public policy in the last analysis."[16] And as Holmes said on another occasion: "General propositions do not decide concrete cases. The decision would depend on a judgment or intuition more subtle than any articulate major premises."[17]

Every case involves an unexpressed major premise. For example, the rules on criminal responsibility and competency to be executed serve to temper the severity of punishment; the rule on competency to stand trial provides pretrial detention or indeterminate confinement; and the rule on testamentary capacity prevents disherison of needy members of a family. These concepts are very much litigation artifacts. The courts grope to find a means of applying the relatively inarticulate standard. More often than not, the rules on procedure are used to govern the outcome of a case.

The lawyer is an advocate; what he says is not evidence; he must present witnesses or documents. Like the host on the television talk show, his job is to get someone else to talk. His task is to furnish the court, and provide for the record, justification or support for a decision, even when it is only something the judge can hang his hat on. Psychiatric testimony generally serves this purpose.[18]

The question is whether the court should use other evidence in the place of psychiatric testimony. Henri Charrière of *Papillon* fame wondered why the prosecutor spent all those plodding years to educate himself, spending all those nights on Roman codes, learning Greek and Latin, just to send him to jail! Would Papillon, though, have preferred an unlearned prosecutor? Is it preferable that a prosecutor not be familiar with Greek, philosophy, or psychiatry? Likewise, would it be preferable that the court rely entirely on lay witnesses rather than on psychiatrists or other experts?[19]

NOTES

1. Frank, J. *Courts on Trial.* P. 91. Under executive privilege, which is ordained in both statute and court decision, much information may be unavailable. In 1789, the Congress enacted a statute (now 5 U.S.C. §22) which authorizes the "heads of each Department" to prescribe "regulations" for the government of their Departments including "the custody, use, and preservation of the records, papers, and property appertaining to it." These regulations have the force of law under this statute. The right of the Executive to impose secrecy is also explicitly recognized in the Freedom of Information Act of 1966. [*Epstein v. Resor*, 296 F. Supp. 214 (N.D. Cal. 1969); noted in *Harv. L. Rev.* 83:928, 1970.] However, in *United States v. Reynolds*, 345 U.S. 1 (1953), a tort action against the Government by widows of civilians killed in the crash of an Air Force plane, the Court inquired into the justification for classifying the Government's report of its investigation of the crash upon plaintiffs' motion to discover it under the Federal Rules of Civil Procedure. Discovery, though, was denied because the report discussed "Top Secret" military equipment which had been on the plane. See Schlesinger, A. Executive Privilege: A Murky History. *Wall Street J.*, March 30, 1973, p. 6.
2. Jurors on the other hand, regardless of their competence, are forced to make an involuntary financial sacrifice, and because they are a cheap resource, their time is abused. In *Barnes v. Boatmen's Nat. Bank*, 384 Mo. 1032, 156 S.W.2d 597 (1941), a contingent fee contract was utilized by a party-litigant who, in contesting a will, employed a psychiatrist whose fee was to be contingent upon the outcome of the case. In a dispute over payment, the court upheld the contract over objection that it was against public policy because it encouraged perjured testimony. See Bomer, H. L. The Compensation of Expert Witnesses. *Law & Contemp. Prob.* 2:510, 1935; Porterfield, P. L. Right to Subpoena Expert Testimony. *Hastings L.J.* 5:50, 1953; Notes, Expert Witness Fees: Protection for the Indigent Party. *Nw. U.L. Rev.* 48:106, 1953; Involuntary Expert Witnesses. *Brooklyn L. Rev.* 13:216, 1947.
3. Beckwith, E. R., and Soberheim, R. Amicus Curiae—Minister of Justice, *Ford L. Rev.* 17:38, 1946; Harper, F. V., and Etherington, E. D. Lobbyists Before the Court. *U. Pa. L. Rev.* 101:1172, 1953; Krislov, S. The Amicus Curiae Brief: From Friendship to Advocacy. *Yale L.J.* 72:694, 1963. With the exception of governmental units which can file amicus briefs as a matter of right, one desiring to file must obtain the consent of all parties or file a motion describing his interest in the case and showing that the brief will cover matter not presented, or inadequately presented by the parties. [28 U.S.C. §1706.] A study of the role of amicus curiae was conducted in 1972 by the Committee on Legal Approaches to Mental Health of the American Orthopsychiatric Association, consisting of Judge Luther Alverson, Mr. Bernard D. Fischman, Dr. Leila Foster, Mr. Charles R. Halpern, Dr. Jay Katz, Mr. Simon Rosenzweig, and Ralph Slovenko, chairman.

4. In the leading case of *Schmerber v. California*, 384 U.S. 757 (1966), the defendant was compelled to give a blood test against his will in a drunk-driving prosecution. Tracing the development of the law, the Supreme Court held that this did not violate the defendant's constitutional rights, noting that "The distinction which has emerged, often expressed in different ways, is that the privilege [against self-incrimination] is a bar against compelling 'communications' or 'testimony,' but that compulsion which makes a suspect or an accused the source of 'real or physical evidence' does not violate it." Thus, the privilege is no bar to compelling the defendant to submit to such tests as fingerprinting, photographing, urine analysis. *State v. Tarrance*, 252 La. 396, 211 So.2d 304 (1968)—defendant was compelled to give a handwriting sample. See also Notes, *Conn. B.J.* 41:125, 1967; *Ohio S. L.J.* 28:185, 1967; *Washburn L.J.* 7:127, 1967.
5. *People v. Stevens*, 194 N.W.2d 370 (Mich. 1972). The Supreme Court in its controversial decision in *Miranda* in 1966 ruled that persons suspected of crime must be advised of their rights before interrogation or their confessions may not be used in court. See Davidson, H. A. Psychiatric Examination and Civil Rights. In Slovenko, R. (Ed.). *Crime, Law and Corrections*. P. 459; Comment, Pretrial Psychiatric Examination and the Privilege against Self-Incrimination. *J. Ill. L. For.* 1971:232.
6. Menninger, K. A. Letter to Editor, *Newsletter of Psychology-Law Soc.*, April 1971, pp. 3–4.
7. Menninger, K. A. *The Crime of Punishment*. P. 138.
8. Oscar K. Diamond Award Address; reported in *Psychiatr. News*, Feb. 16, 1972, p. 27.
9. Woodruff, W. A. Letter to Editor. *Med. Trib.*, Dec. 1, 1971, p. 11.
10. Advisory Committee's Notes to Rule 706, *Proposed Rules of Evidence for the U.S. District Courts and Magistrates* (March 1971).
11. Erikson, E. The Ontogeny of Ritualization; presented in June 1965 to the Royal Society as a contribution to a symposium on "Ritualization in Animals and in Man."
12. For an inventory of proverbs, see Wilson, F. P. *Dictionary of English Proverbs*. New York: Oxford, 1970.
13. Cooney, J. E. Rising Courtroom Use of Expert Witnesses Creates Controversy. *Wall Street J.*, April 20, 1971, p. 1.
14. Goldsmith, S. R., and Mandell, A. J. The Psychodynamic Formulation: A Critique of a Psychiatric Ritual. *Am. J. Psychiatry* 125:1738, 1969. See also Chapman, L. P., and J. P. Genesis of Popular but Erroneous Psychodiagnostic Observations. *J. Abnorm. Psychol.* 72:193, 1967.
15. Pasamanick B., Dinitz, S., and Lafton, N. Psychiatric Orientation and Its Relation to Diagnosis and Treatment in a Mental Hospital. *Am. J. Psychiatry* 116:127, 1959. See also Arnhoff, F. N. Some Factors Influencing the Unreliability of Clinical Judgments. *J. Clin. Psychol.* 10:272, 1954; Dymond, R. F. Can Clinicians Predict Individual Behavior? *J. Pers.* 22:151, 1953; Mehlman, B. The Reliability of Psychiatric Diagnoses. *J. Abnorm. Soc. Psychol.* 47:577, 1952; Zigler, E., and Phillips, L. Psychiatric Diagnosis: A Critique. *J. Abnorm. Soc. Psychol.* 3:607, 1961.
16. Holmes, O. W. *The Common Law*. Boston: Little, Brown, 1881. Pp. 35–36.
17. *Lochner v. New York*, 198 U.S. 45, 76 (1905).
18. The law's use of social science, in general, is discussed in Cairns, H. *Law and the Social Sciences*. New York: Harcourt, Brace, 1935; Jones, H. W. (Ed.). *Law and the Social Role of Science*. New York: Rockefeller University Press, 1966; Rosen, P. L. *The Supreme Court and Social Science*. Urbana: University of Illinois Press, 1972; Stone, J. *Law and the Social Sciences: The Second Half Century*. Minneapolis: University of Minnesota Press, 1966; Clark, K. B. The Desegregation Cases: Criticism of the Social Scientist's Role. *Vill. L. Rev.* 5:224, 1960; Geis, G. The Social Sciences and the Law. *U. Wash. L. Rev.* 1:569, 1962; Greenberg, G. Social Scientists Take the Stand: A Review and

Appraisal of Their Testimony in Litigation. *Mich. L. Rev.* 54:953, 1956; Hazard, G. C. Limitations on the Uses of Behavioral Science in the Law. *Case W. Res. L. Rev.* 19:71, 1967; Kaplan, A. Behavioral Science and the Law. *Case W. Res. L. Rev.* 19:57, 1967; Katz, M. The Unmasking of Dishonest Pretensions: Toward an Interpretation of the Role of Social Science in Constitutional Litigation. *Am. Sociologist* 6:54, 1971; Loevinger, L. Law and Science as Rival Systems. *U. Fla. L. Rev.* 19:530, 1966; Maslow, W. How Social Scientists Can Shape Legal Process. *Vill. L. Rev.* 5:241, 1960; Nagel, S. S. Law and the Social Sciences: What Can Social Science Contribute? *J.A.B.A.* 51:356, 1965; Pope, J. The Presentation of Scientific Evidence. *Texas L. Rev.* 31:794, 1953; Riesman, D. Some Observations on Law and Psychology. *U. Chi. L. Rev.* 19:30, 1951; Simpson, S. P., and Field, R. Law and the Social Sciences. *Va. L. Rev.* 32:855, 1946; Touster, S. Law and Psychology. *Am. Behav. Sci.* 5:3, 1961.

19. In the eighteenth century, Franz Gall introduced the theory of phrenology, which related a person's mental faculties to the conformation of his skull. In the notable trial of the pirate Tardy, his bumps of combativeness and acquisitiveness were adjudged larger than his bump of veneration. [Slovenko, R. A History of Criminal Procedures as Related to Mental Disorders. *Psychoanal. Rev.* 55:223, 1968; revised version, *W. Va. L. Rev.* 71:135, 1969.] A 19th-century poster, exhibited recently at the New York Cultural Center, certifies to the qualifications of a phrenologist.

A FREE LECTURE!

PHRENOLOGY!

DELIVERED BY WILLIAM CARROLL

January 5, 1860

Each lecture will close with the public examination of the heads of two individuals chosen by the audience.

Examinations daily at his room, with verbal or written descriptions of character.

From O. S. and L. N. Fowler TO THE PUBLIC

This is to certify that the bearer, William Carroll, has taken a full course of lessons calculated to prepare him for teaching and practicing the science of Phrenology, Physiology, and Anatomy. That he is also still farther prepared for this profession by an ardent love of the sciences and by excellent natural capabilities for that purpose; to a clear mind and good talents for learning, he adds good speaking capabilities and a phrenological organization adapting him to make an excellent examiner and lecturer. Our friends and the public may rely on obtaining from him a correct, reliable and thorough delineation of their characters. To these natural gifts he adds a lofty, noble, aspiring ambition; a good moral and strictly conscientious tone; good taste, and an organism which will wear well and improve with age. Nature has done more for him than for most persons. We commend him to the public patronage and confidence.

Subscriptions received for the
Phrenological and Water Cure Journals, and Life Illustrated

The Examination of Heads

12 ½ cents
children half-price
a reduction made for families and schools
November 15, 1853

3. WITNESSES AND THE CREDIBILITY OF TESTIMONY

THE primitive method of settling disputed matters was by fist or club. Witnesses obviously played no role in such settlements. Gradually, the concept of a trial evolved with its concomitant rules regarding the competency of witnesses and the admissibility of evidence. The early method of deciding disputes, however, has influenced the development of the rules of procedure; within this evolving framework various psychological notions are being used to assess the credibility of testimony.

Historically, litigation is a substitute for trial by ordeal or by battle. During the feudal period, the issue in important cases, such as a disputed claim to land or an accusation of unjustifiable homicide, was generally determined by judicial combat between the principals or their legally appointed champions rather than in a courtroom. In knightly array, the two fought it out and the vanquished, if still alive, suffered whatever penalty the law prescribed.[1]

Around A.D. 1100, ambitious princes took heed of the political systems of Athens and republican Rome and adopted many of the same concepts in order to support and expand their jurisdiction. The function of the jury at this time was to give support to the king's administrative officials and, later, to his traveling justices in their efforts to extend the jurisdiction of the king's courts throughout England. The strong men of the locality were drawn to the aid of the judges and, as the jury, were not only witnesses but a determining body. These functions were not split as they are today between our modern jury and witnesses; rather these men had, or were supposed to have had, information regarding the matters in issue.[2] It is interesting to note that the original meaning of the word *juror* is one who took an oath and swore to declare truly what he knew or believed in a given case. There were no rules concerning the way in which the jurors acquired their knowledge.[3] During this period the independent witness was thought of as a meddler and, if he intervened, was in peril of being held guilty of maintenance.

The advent of the modern witness took place in the sixteenth century, the time of the end of the feudal order. Disputes were no longer provincial matters, and the jury gained in importance, becoming a symbol of political freedom. The Elizabethan Act of 1562, which created the statutory offense of perjury and provided for compulsory attendance of witnesses, initiated a new epoch in the law of evidence. Thereafter, the facts of the case were presented by outside witnesses and not by members of the jury. Previously the jurors were to know everything about the case, now they were to know nothing. The *tabula rasa* dictum, soon to be current in philosophy, found judicial application.

Initially, however, these outside witnesses were received with some circumspection as possible perjurers, and if there was any reason to suspect that a witness might be inclined to lie, he was considered incompetent to testify.[4] The common law borrowed heavily from the canon law in designating certain persons as incompetent to serve as witnesses. Holdsworth in his *History of English Law* points out:

> The canon law rejected the testimony of all males under fourteen and females under twelve, of the blind and the deaf and the dumb, of slaves, of infamous persons, and those convicted of crime, of excommunicated persons, of poor persons, and of women in criminal cases, of persons connected with either party by consanguinity and affinity, or belonging to the household of either party, of the enemies of either party, and of Jews, heretics, and pagans.[5]

The grounds of incompetency, as developed through the centuries, have been broadly categorized under five I's:

1. Interest: a witness, whether or not a party to the controversy, if pecuniarily interested in the outcome of the cause, was not allowed to testify because of the temptation to falsify.

2. Insanity: a person considered insane was thought not to have the mental capacity to testify.

3. Infancy: a child was considered incompetent to understand the nature of an oath or to narrate with understanding the facts of what he had seen.

4. Infidelity: a person who did not believe in a Supreme Being who was a rewarder of truth and an avenger of falsehood was deemed incapable of taking an oath and therefore of testifying.

5. Infamy: part of the punishment for crime in early common law was to render the guilty person infamous and, among other sanctions, he lost the right to testify in a court of law.

In addition, a wife was not permitted to testify for or against her husband because in theory husband and wife were one (and that one was the husband).

A number of general basic reforms in trial procedure were accomplished during the seventeenth century, and major reforms also occurred during the nineteenth century, in a large measure stimulated by the writings of Charles Dickens. Today the rules on competency of witnesses have been replaced with the general principle that any person of "proper understanding" is a competent witness. The rules on competency have been converted into rules of credibility whereby nearly every proposed witness is allowed to testify, but on cross-examination his credibility may be impeached.[6] The question of competency, when raised, is a preliminary matter for the trial judge, whereas, once the witness is allowed to testify, his credibility is a question for the jury.

Cross-examination includes the right, as the courts say, "to place the witness in his proper setting and put the weight of his testimony and his credibility to a test, without which the jury cannot fairly appraise them." The credibility of the witness is always relevant in the search for truth. The main lines of attack upon the credibility of a witness are: (1) by showing that the witness on a previous occasion has made statements inconsistent with his present testimony; (2) by specific contradiction, proving that some statement of fact made by the witness is in fact otherwise; (3) by showing that the witness is biased by reason of such influences as kinship with one party or hostility to another, or motives of pecuniary interest, legitimate or corrupt; (4) by showing a defect of capacity in the witness to observe, remember, or recount the matters testified about; (5) by attacking the character of the witness; and (6) by showing that the witness lacks the religious belief which would give the fullest traditional sanction to his obligation to speak the truth (now obsolete).

Unquestionably, judges or juries are swayed by the relative attractiveness or unattractiveness of plaintiff or defendant or of the witnesses. As a consequence, cross-examination sometimes ends up being a smearing rather than a discrediting process.

THE RULES OF EVIDENCE AND THE ROLE OF PSYCHIATRY

The rules of evidence, including the method of challenging credibility, may appear to be an affront to common sense, but, as Chief Justice Vanderbilt once remarked, "The entire history of the law of evidence has been marked by a continuous search for more rational rules, first as to competency of witnesses, and then as to the admissibility of evidence."[7] Courts frequently point out that the rules of evidence, designed to obtain the truth, are intended to exclude unreliable testimony, such as hearsay, and false and dishonest testimony.

The legal ban on opinion testimony and the admonition to tell the

whole truth and nothing but the truth are designed to rule out gratui-
tous imagination and conjecture. While by "truth" the law seems to
accept a naive correspondence theory of language and reality, the adversary system is actually based on the proposition that a human being does
not and cannot behave as a mere "dataphone"; conditions for knowing
include memory and perception, feeling and will, attention and thought.
Selectivity, inherent in the process of knowing (well depicted in the
Japanese film *Rashomon*), is theoretically leveled out by the presentation of viewpoints under the adversary system. The dialectic of opposites,
which obtains in an adversarial proceeding, brings forth a new truth.

The concept of the Anglo-American system is that truth is best dis-
cerned by application of the rules of evidence in an adversarial proceeding, a procedure well suited to the popular American conditioning to
games. The witness may feel that he goes through an ordeal just as
harrowing as the ancient ordeal by battle. In various ways the witness
is placed under stress as it is believed that this will aid in the ascertainment of truth, whether the witness be shy or bold. The unfamiliar courtroom procedure and legal language are built-in stress factors. At one
time, and still in most countries, the witness had to stand (from which
derives the term *witness stand*), which increased his anxiety. The witness
must swear to tell the truth, and he may be subjected to a vigorous cross-
examination.[8] Members of the bench and bar frequently say that "cross-
examination of a witness is one of the principal and most efficacious
tests which the law has devised for the discovery of truth."[9]

In the courtroom setting, what role does the psychiatrist or psychologist have to play in the search for truth? One psychologist observes:

> When a reader comes upon a statement in the introductory pages of a
> psychological test, as he frequently may, that one of the practical applica-
> tions of psychological science is the evaluation of testimony, he readily
> accepts the statement as true and reads quickly on, with a quiet glow of satis-
> faction that science is such an aid in the search for truth and justice. Al-
> though it is true that psychology can and should render such service to
> society, it is an unfortunate paradox that so little has been actually ac-
> complished. There is a surprising lack of work in this area.[10]

That there is need for a better test in the search for truth is well illustrated in the unsound psychological notion expressed, for example, by
one trial judge—"wiping hands during testimony is almost always an
indication of lying."[11] In the years preceding World War I, there was
considerable interest in Europe, especially in Germany, in the psychology of testimony. Sigmund Freud in 1906 delivered a lecture to a law

class at the University of Vienna entitled "Psycho-analysis and the Ascertaining of Truth in Courts of Law" in which he said:

There is a growing recognition of the untrustworthiness of statements
made by witnesses, at present the basis of so many judgments in Courts of
Law; and this has quickened in all of you, who are to become judges and
advocates, an interest in a new method of investigation, the purpose of
which is to lead the accused person to establish his own guilt or innocence
objectively. This method is of a psychological and experimental character
and is based upon psychological research; it is closely connected with certain
views which have only recently been propounded in medical psychology.[12]

The task of the therapist, Freud said, is the same as the task of the
judge: he must discover the hidden psychic material. "To do this," Freud
said, "we have invented various methods of detection, some of which
lawyers are now going to imitate." However, Freud cautioned: "It is
necessary to consider [the] points of difference in the psychological situation in the two cases."[13]

Was Freud, while cautious, naive in his assumption that psychoanalysis has something to offer in ascertaining truth in courts?[14] Although
Freud failed his examination in medical jurisprudence—his only failure
—he was a genius and generally was not naive about the law. At one
time he seriously considered the study of law instead of medicine, perhaps because of the discrimination and persecution that he himself en-
dured. When, in 1938, he was exiled from his country, he carried a
manuscript on Moses, the supreme law-giver of the Jewish people. He was
intensely interested in law and criminal behavior, but apart from his lecture on psychoanalysis and the ascertainment of truth, he was exceed-
ingly pessimistic about the possible application of psychoanalysis to the
legal process.[15]

Shortly after Freud's lecture, in 1908, Hugo Munsterberg, Professor
of Psychology at Harvard, in a book entitled *On the Witness Stand*,
suggested that prospective witnesses should be tested for reliability in
experimental situations before their testimony be accepted in court. He
severely criticized the legal profession for its failure to apply psychological principles to the evaluation of testimony.[16]

Dean John Wigmore, whose name is synonymous with the law of evidence, quickly took Munsterberg to task. In an article satirically cast in
the form of a lawsuit against Munsterberg for defamation of the legal
profession, Wigmore asked: "[W]here are the exact and precise experimental and psychological methods of ascertaining and measuring the
testimonial certitude of witnesses and the guilty consciousness of ac-

cused persons?" Tell us, Wigmore urged, about the methods that might be applicable to judicial practice. Wigmore pleaded ignorance to the exactness and practical utility of these wonderful methods, which the legal profession had persisted in rejecting or ignoring.[17]

The Hiss Trial

Not until the spectacular Hiss trial of the early 1950s did the issue of psychiatric evaluation of a witness again attract much attention.[18] Alger Hiss, Chairman of the Carnegie Foundation for Peace and the fair-haired boy of the Democratic party, was accused by Whittaker Chambers of passing secrets to Communists in the 1930s. The fate of the Democratic party was at stake, Senator Joe McCarthy having charged it with twenty years of treason. The defense offered psychiatric testimony designed to impeach the credibility of the government witness, Whittaker Chambers. Judge Goddard, ruling the psychiatric testimony admissible, said:

> It is apparent that the outcome of this trial is dependent, to a great extent, upon the testimony of one man—Whittaker Chambers. Mr. Chambers' credibility is one of the major issues upon which the jury must pass. The opinion of the jury—formed upon their evaluation of all the evidence laid before them—is the decisive authority on this question, as on all questions of fact. The existence of insanity or mental derangement is admissible for the purpose of discrediting a witness. Evidence of insanity is not merely for the judge on the preliminary question of competency but goes to the jury to affect credibility.

Dr. Carl Binger, psychiatrist, testified that Chambers was a "psychopath with a tendency toward making false accusations." Binger testified that his first opinion was based on "personal observation of Mr. Chambers at the first trial for five days and one day at this trial" and that "he had read plays, poems, articles, and book reviews by Mr. Chambers and books he had translated from German."

On cross-examination, Binger's testimony was discredited. As so often happens, a fabric is made to look meaningless when every fiber is scrutinized. The forest is lost for the trees. Binger on direct examination had pointed out Chambers' untidiness, and on cross-examination he was made to acknowledge that the trait was found in such persons as Albert Einstein, Heywood Broun, Will Rogers, Owen D. Young, Bing Crosby, and Thomas A. Edison. Binger testified that Chambers habitually gazed at the ceiling while testifying and seemed to have no direct relation with his examiner. The prosecutor in a turnabout told Binger: "We have made a count of the number of times you looked at the ceiling. During the first ten minutes you looked at the ceiling nineteen times; in the next fifteen minutes you looked up twenty times, for the next fifteen minutes ten times, and for the last fifteen minutes ten times more. We counted a total of fifty-nine times that you looked at the ceiling in fifty minutes. Now I was wondering whether that was any symptom of a psychopathic personality?" Shifting uneasily in the witness chair, Binger replied, "Not alone." Binger had testified that stealing was a psychopathic symptom and the prosecutor asked him: "Did you ever take a hotel towel or Pullman towel?" Binger replied, "I can't swear whether I did or not, I don't think so." The prosecutor thereupon asked: "And if any member of this jury had stolen a towel, would that be evidence of a psychopathic personality?"

Would you have believed Whittaker Chambers? The jury did. Until December 12, 1958, he was senior editor of *Time* earning $30,000 a year. His family, however, had no social or community ties. His grandmother, who went around the house brandishing a carving knife, was put in an asylum; his grandfather was an alcoholic; his father was unfaithful to his mother; his brother committed suicide; and Whittaker himself made an unsuccessful attempt at "self-execution" (his own label) prior to the first Hiss trial. Binger gave his opinion after listening to a seventy-minute hypothetical question "that accentuated unpalatable aspects of Mr. Chambers' life."[19]

Fifteen years later, Binger, reflecting on the *Hiss* case, had this to say:

My opinion of Chambers and the Hiss trial was based almost entirely on the seven volumes of sworn testimony which he deposed in Baltimore before the trial. This was an exposition of a life so irregular and so delinquent that one could only interpret it as the story of a psychopath. Many of my psychiatric friends agreed with me in this decision, but were less willing to expose themselves to ridicule and contumely than I was. Perhaps they were wiser. But I never regretted my stand nor had I any serious doubts about Hiss's innocence. I did suspect some hidden, unconscious relationship with Chambers, of which I believe Hiss was unaware, and that this led him into an involvement which might well have looked like a conspiracy. He certainly never gave signed state documents to Chambers. . . . The prosecutor, Mr. Murphy, who looked like a dumb cop, turned out to be highly astute and tricky. He resorted to all kinds of subterfuges to trip me up. He tried to turn words around in my mouth and forced me to answer "yes" and "no" to questions framed by him in such a manner that the answers did not convey the meaning that I wished to present. I know that this is all part of the game, but it seemed to me shocking and preposterous. I had only one wish and that was to tell the truth and not lose my temper. I think I did both. Mr. Murphy, on the other hand, was determined to try to have me lose my temper and to distort the truth.[20]

COMPETENCY OF PSYCHIATRY IN ASSESSING CREDIBILITY

Where do we go from here? According to orthodox doctrine, proof of character in assessing credibility is limited to reputation evidence. For example, the *California Code of Civil Procedure*, applicable to criminal as well as civil trials, specifies: "[A] witness may be impeached by the party against whom he was called . . . by evidence that his general reputation for truth, honesty, or integrity is bad, but not by evidence of particular wrongful acts except that it may be shown by the examination of the witness, or the record of the judgment, that he had been convicted of a felony."

Should evidence of character in assessing credibility pass from the "crucible of the community" to the "couch of the psychiatrist"?[21] The question today is most frequently raised in sex-offense cases where the credibility of the accused or the prosecuting witness is in question. The victim frequently is a child of such early age that the report often cannot be considered reliable. In other cases, both the accused and the prosecuting witness may contend that they have a good reputation for morality in the community and that they are beyond "lewd lascivious conduct." Often a vindictive or rejected person may want to hurt the ex-friend by involving him in a legal procedure. The *Model Code of Evidence*, adopted in some states, allows not only reputation evidence but also opinion evidence as to the character of the accused in a criminal action. This rule makes it clear that the belief of a character witness whose conclusion as to the accused's character is based on personal acquaintance rather than on reputation will not be excluded.

Is psychiatry capable of devising a test which can measure credibility? Test results of so-called lie detectors, truth serum, and drunkometers are uniformly rejected by the courts. Dr. Henry Davidson, psychiatrist, asserts that psychiatrists can play a major role in the administration of justice by appraising the credibility of witnesses.[22] There is a strong emotional component in the motivation and memory of witnesses, Davidson says, and thus credibility represents an area that should fall within the special field of the psychiatrist. Observation is selective and in large part dependent upon the condition of the observer as well as upon inner motivations. To give effective and accurate testimony, a witness must observe intelligently, remember clearly, speak coherently, and be free of any emotional drive to distort the truth. According to Davidson, the analysis of these traits should be a job for the psychiatrist.

The major clinical conditions affecting testimonial capacity, Davidson says, are psychosis, mental deficiency, drug addiction, alcoholism, personality disorders, certain organic involvements of the brain, and sometimes certain forms of psychoneurosis. The schizophrenic person can report an event with carbon-paper fidelity, but may make an unreliable witness because of defective observation, distorted memory processes, or paranoid ideas. A senile psychotic person is unreliable as a witness because of frequent delusions of infidelity, impairment of memory, and delusions of ingratitude. The hypomanic witness is dangerous because his speech is plausible and positive; but, as every psychiatrist knows, the things he says can be the stuff of which dreams are made. The drug addict may not be a good witness because he may be under the toxic influence of a drug, or his testimony may not be reliable because the issue happens to concern his source of supply. The mental defective may make an adequate witness if the event is one that can be described simply; but since most events are complex, involving many subtle details, the defective would make a poor witness because of his deficient powers of observation and his inability to paint a vivid verbal picture. The alcoholic is often at the mercy of mixed and unpredictable emotions; the memory defects of chronic alcoholics are well known to psychiatrists. The psychopath will twist his tongue to say anything. Among psychoneurotics, recessional states or depressive reactions may result in distorted interpretations of events.[23]

A paranoid patient, if not deteriorated, may appear to talk sense, but his testimony may be part of the delusional network. The late Ralph S. Banay, psychiatrist, said:

> The problem of the paranoid personality offers an illustrative example of the usefulness of psychiatric testimony, especially in civil cases. Paranoids, who have a marked proclivity for getting into legal difficulties, often make a favorable appearance in court when not crossed or agitated, and they may impress the untrained observer as rational and sincere. They could conceivably mislead a judge, an attorney, or a jury into the sincerity of their claim, but they would less likely deceive a clinically experienced psychiatrist. Similarly, in many borderline cases or in maladies of obscure manifestation, the root of the trouble may be discernible to the clinician although it is hidden from other observers.[24]

One law writer believes that psychiatric diagnosis, whether based on clinical examination or courtroom observation alone, should be admitted whenever it is offered to show the unreliability of a witness. He suggests that the psychiatrist sit with a cross-examining attorney, at the counsel table, and thus "direct the cross-examination, thereby approximating a personal interview with the witness."[25]

In the courtroom the psychiatrist may observe the witness's mood, pressure of talk, stream of thought, brightness, content of thinking, memory. But in the courtroom, where nobody believes anybody, the aura of cross-examination, with its concomitant implication of hostility and adversity of interest, provides an emotional climate far different from that of the ideal psychiatric interview. The witness feels attacked and abused, which immediately elicits defense mechanisms that can only shut out or distort pertinent psychiatric material.[26]

In the often-cited case of *State v. Driver*, decided in 1921, a twelve-year-old girl, upon whom an attempted rape was allegedly committed, was called as a witness. The defendant offered to show by the testimony of a psychiatrist that the girl was a moral pervert and not trustworthy. On the basis of courtroom observation, the expert was prepared to testify that he would classify the girl as a lying moron and unworthy of belief. The evidence was designed to be an attack upon her truthfulness, aimed at her credibility; and the inference to be drawn from the testimony, if it had been permitted, would have been that she was a habitual and confirmed liar because of her mental defectiveness. The court refused to hear the proffered evidence and said:

[A] person's knowledge of an assailed witness's reputation, gained alone from what has been said against him on the trial, or from his conduct on the trial, is not sufficient to render him competent as a character witness. It was attempted to make the expert competent by showing that he had partially heard the evidence, had observed the girl on the stand, and concluded that she was a moron of the class of liars, and hence unworthy of belief. We are not convinced that the time-honored and well settled and undefined rule of impeachment of the veracity of a witness should be thus innovated upon. It is yet to be demonstrated that psychological and medical tests are practical and will detect a lie on the witness stand.[27]

To vary the facts in *Driver*, consider the case of a woman in her late twenties who had a very poor childhood relationship with her father. Although rather attractive, she dated rarely and never married. She meets a man at a social gathering, and following some pleasant conversation, he offers to take her home. She accepts, but he drives to a secluded spot. She reports that her memory was a "complete blank" from that time until she recalls finding herself in his arms. Let us assume that she regularly sees a psychiatrist and on the day following the alleged incident, she sees him and, still in a very anxious and overwrought condition, she tells him that she was raped. If this event becomes the subject of prosecution, does the psychiatrist have probative evidence to offer unavailable to others? The psychiatrist knows her to be a hysterical woman who regularly mixes fact with fantasy, but he is also aware that hysterical women are not immune from rape.[28]

A psychiatrist may not be able to detect a lie on the witness stand, but is he able to detect it when the witness has talked over the matter with him in psychotherapy? Theodor Reik, in his book *The Unknown Murderer*, says that psychoanalysis has no contribution to make to evidence of guilt, as it is concerned with mental (inner) reality rather than material (outer) reality. A therapist does not ordinarily check on material reality. He is ordinarily concerned with the patient's view of the world rather than with what the world actually is. He does not cross-question the patient. Some therapists say that outside information about the patient interferes with their clinical work, and they prefer to close their eyes to it. They know the situation only through the eyes of the patient. Something more, then, is needed to test veracity.

Reliability of Testimony

Who, then, is reliable? Children are not terribly reliable. Mental defectives are not reliable. People with organic brain disease are not reliable. Psychotics are not reliable. Psychopaths are liars. Obsessive compulsives deny various things and obviously cannot be very reliable about these things.

The law, with its emphasis on structure, is replacing the old categories whereby large groups of people were excluded as incompetent (those involved in the five I's of interest, insanity, infancy, infidelity, and infamy) with psychiatric categories. Popular disapproval of drug addiction and chronic alcoholism is so strong that it would be imprudent to introduce an addict as a witness. The courts say: "The habitual use of opium is known to utterly deprave the victim of its use and render him unworthy of belief."[29] "We believe it will be admitted that habitual users of opium, or other like narcotics, become notorious liars. The habit of lying comes doubtless from the fact that these narcotics users pass the greater part of their life in an unreal world, and thus become unable to distinguish between images and facts, between illusion and realities."[30]

A minority of courts take the position that addicts *per se* are predilected toward untruthfulness and, by so holding, the court takes away the jury's prerogative to assess credibility.[31] In an old parallel, St. Thomas maintained, with the authority of St. Chrysostom, *Daemoni,*

Etiam Vera Dicenti, Non Est Credendum (the devil is not to be believed, even when he tells the truth). In the absence of other proofs, it was said, one must not proceed against those who are accused by devils. Christ imposed silence on the demons when they spoke the truth.

Obviously, though, no one can judge the reliability of a group of people as a class. It may be expeditious, but a great error, to generalize. For example, it is sometimes said that a person is an alcoholic and then his testimony is excluded on the ground that alcoholics are not reliable witnesses. However, many persons are alcoholics (or have an alcoholic problem) even if they have not drunk any alcohol in a year or more. Many who have an alcoholic problem hold most responsible positions and are reliable when not drinking to excess. If all alcoholics were disqualified as reliable observers, we should disqualify many judges, lawyers, psychiatrists, and clergymen. But suppose, instead of deciding on the basis of class, we consider each individual as an individual, try to understand his reactions to various situations, and examine the reliability of his stories under various circumstances. Would that be of any help in resolving disputes?

To estimate one's reliability supposedly calls for knowing something of his unconscious motivation. Lawyers are specialists in verbal communication and usually deal with conscious motivation, but psychiatrists, specialized in listening with the third ear, are concerned about unconscious motivation and nonverbal communication. Of course, lawyers such as Perry Mason read between the lines, understanding unconscious motivation though not identifying it as such.

On a practical, if personal, level we all have known friends who are not alcoholic or addictive or psychopathic, but when they make out their federal income tax return, it becomes very questionable how far they are reliable. There may be times when perhaps no one is reliable. On the other hand, there are individuals who list every conceivable item on their tax return. They are scrupulously honest. We might say that they are reliable honest people. But the psychiatrist looks behind the scene and asks, "Why does this person have to be so honest?" Hamlet, looking behind his mother's pretenses, said: "The lady doth protest too much, me thinks." When somebody is too scrupulously honest, he may be worried about his dishonest tendencies and distrustful of himself. An individual may be very compulsive, a perfectionist, always being sure that he is clean, et cetera, but when we look carefully at him, we may find that underneath his clean shirt, he has not bathed or wears dirty underwear.

RELATIONSHIP OF MAN'S BIOGRAPHY AND HIS MESSAGE

What is the relationship of man to his message? Philosophy traditionally has taught that words lead an independent life. Under the
correspondence theory of truth, the relation studied is strictly that
between the statement and the world. Personalizing is ruled out under
the well-known ad hominem objection. But, we may ask, does the ad
hominem (or ad feminam) objection need reevaluation? What is the
relationship between ideas, mentation, and biography? A person gains
in understanding his own philosophy and ideas by examination and
analysis of his mental processes and motivations, as psychoanalysis may
attest. Do we likewise, in examining the philosophy or message of another person, add a dimension to it by understanding his personality?
Man's message reveals the man; does man reveal the message?[32]

Freud, although never concealing his condition as a Jew, often worried about protecting his new science from a closeness with the personality of its creator. Notwithstanding, psychoanalysis is often called a
"Jewish science." David Bakan in his book, *Freud and the Jewish Mysti-
cal Tradition*, says that Freudianism is a laic transformation of the Jewish mystique. Bakan shows the decisive importance of Freud's Jewishness
in the formulation of his work and the need to be aware of this fact for
the best interpretation of his work.

That Immanuel Kant's neighbors set their clocks by his routine is not
surprising to one having knowledge of his obsessive behavior. Schopen-
hauer too is known to have been an obsessional neurotic. Jean Jacques
Rousseau's noble savage and state-of-nature philosophy may be linked
with his psychosexual infantilism, which expressed itself also in exhibi-
tionism, narcissism, and homosexual trends. Bishop Berkeley's idealism
and denial of reality may be tied in with his attitudes regarding excre-
tion. Nietzsche's mother was considered to be hereditarily tainted.
Hegel's philosophical system begins where repression is involved, where
thesis turns into antithesis. Albert Deutsch in his book, *The Mentally Ill
in America*, raises the issue of the credibility of Mrs. E. P. W. Packard,
the famous crusader for the enactment of commitment laws; he points to
her childhood institutionalization at the Worcester State Hospital and
to the psychiatric history that showed at one time she claimed to be the
Mother of Christ and the Third Person of the Blessed Trinity.

Is such biography helpful to a study of a message? The roots of psy-
chohistory, as it is called, may go back to Freud's *Leonardo da Vinci:
A Study in Psychosexuality*, published in 1916, which analyzed the
Renaissance genius on the basis of his work and from available records,

and to his work, in 1939, in *Moses and Monotheism,* which attempted to discover in Moses' life the origins of Christianity. Historian Robert G. L. Waite in a postscript in *The Mind of Adolf Hitler* praises Dr. Walter Langer's use in his secret wartime report of psychoanalytic principles to investigate Hitler's psyche. The technique, he says, led not only to predictions of uncanny accuracy but to insights never provided by historians relying on traditional research methods.

It is necessary, it seems, to distinguish the various functions of language—informative, expressive, directive—that is, to transmit information, to express mood, and to promote action. Different criteria are relevant in evaluating each function: truth and falsehood for the informative; sincerity or insincerity, valuable or otherwise, for the expressive; and proper or improper, right or wrong, for the directive. Of all disciplines, there is the fullest exploitation of the genetic dimension in psychoanalysis; psychoanalysis links the present with genesis; but that is for the purpose of treatment. Genesis or biography has little relevance to a person's message if the message is to be evaluated in terms of truth and falsehood. The fact that Kant's neighbors set their clocks by his afternoon walks has no logical bearing upon the truth or informative significance of his philosophy. From his character we may surmise that he would ponder his statements at length, but the psychological origin of a belief, the motive for holding it, and the condition that leads to its acceptance are all irrelevant to its truth or falsehood. Kekulé, the chemist who formulated the benzene ring, dreamed the night before of a snake with its tail in its mouth, but the theory of benzene rings is not to be equated with a dream about a snake. Freud's explanation of how belief in God is born need not be inconsistent with that belief. A message is substantiated by the available evidence, not by its genesis.

If the function of a message, however, is expressive and directive as well as informative (and usually all three functions are included) then, since criteria other than truth and falsehood are involved in its evaluation, biography should be not only helpful but essential to an evaluation and understanding of the message.

The court is essentially concerned with the informative function of a message; and the fact that an individual *may* be an unreliable witness does not imply that he *will* be unreliable. No witness is completely unreliable at all times. The courtroom process is a practical one, however, and when testimony conflicts and the evidence of a witness is crucial, the ad hominem approach may be practically, but not theoretically, justified. There are posters in some libraries which say, "If it is the truth, what does it matter who said it?", but in the mundane world, it is not only what a witness says but how he says it and who he is that is important. This is not epistemology. To look at a man, including his sacroiliac, is justified in terms of convenience and public policy, resulting in a rough sense of justice. It is a question of fair judgment; and it is thought that psychiatry may lend a hand in reaching that judgment. Yet, as pointed out, a number of factors in the legal setting make it difficult, perhaps impossible, to obtain a reliable psychiatric evaluation. A psychiatric evaluation usually rests on the complete trust between the patient and psychiatrist. This trust implies that the psychiatrist is totally on the patient's side, will not reveal information the patient has confided, and will be primarily concerned with the patient's welfare rather than that of society.

The Psychiatrist As Detective

Freud, in his lecture, pointed out that a psychiatrist with a patient is different from a lawyer with a witness. A psychiatrist can allow himself to be hoodwinked, because if the psychiatrist does not show his belief in the patient, he will not be able to establish a successful relationship with him. The patient does not hurt the psychiatrist in hoodwinking him. Rather he is hurting himself. On the witness stand, however, in an attempt to hoodwink, the witness seeks to protect rather than to hurt himself.

A sharp poker player probably knows better than a psychiatrist whether a person is lying or, as the legal test puts it, whether the emotional or mental condition of the witness may affect his ability to tell the truth. A psychiatrist is a doctor, not a lie detector. A lawyer, too, has his shortcomings as an investigator. Although Perry Mason solves cases on the stand (he also solves cases out of court), skillful interrogation and evaluation can more readily take place in the police station than in the courtroom. Such a procedure, however, is against our tradition of law enforcement. In *Leyra v. Denno*, the defendant, after being questioned for the greater part of four days by the state police concerning the murder of his aged parents, complained of an acutely painful sinus attack.[33] Having promised to get him a doctor, the police instead got a psychiatrist with a considerable knowledge of hypnosis. Working in a room that was wired, rather than rendering medical aid, the psychiatrist "by subtle and suggestive questions simply continued the police effort" to obtain a confession. The Supreme Court invalidated the confession and denounced the admission of statements made to the psychiatrist as "so clearly the product of mental coercion that their use as evidence is inconsistent with due process."

It is an open question whether a trial court has the power to order a witness to submit to psychiatric examination; the refusal to order a psychiatric examination has invariably been held not to be an abuse of discretion. When the court does order such examinations, what sanctions does it have available to compel compliance? Rule 35 of the *Federal Rules of Civil Procedure* and similar state statutes authorize trial courts to order a physical or mental examination of a party when his physical or mental condition is in controversy, that is, to determine injury sustained by a party in a personal injury suit. The Rule probably does not include psychiatric examination as to credibility, especially of an ordinary witness, as credibility is not a matter directly in controversy. The power to order a psychiatric examination, although not provided by statute, may be said to be part of inherent or implied judicial power;[34] but even in rape cases some courts have been hesitant to order psychiatric examination of prosecuting females.[35]

Hypnosis is accepted by the American Medical Association as a valid medical technique. It is accepted by both the American Medical Association and the American Psychological Association as a legitimate psychiatric method of inquiry; but its use in the legal process at the pretrial or trial stage is highly dubious. Can greater reliability be gained through hypnotic testimony, despite the danger of increased suggestibility of the hypnotized witness? What is the value of courtroom hypnosis in relation to pretrial hypnosis? The use of hypnosis or sodium amytal (truth serum) by District Attorney Jim Garrison on his star witness in the alleged investigation of President Kennedy's assassination was a national scandal. Shortly before, Dr. Joseph Satten, then of the Menninger Foundation, at the behest of defense counsel, made a videotape of a sodium amytal interview of a person accused of murdering his wife. Its use was allowed at trial, resulting in the exculpation of the accused and was announced in television newscasts as a breakthrough in the search for truth. An Ohio case is one of the few examples of in-court hypnosis (the subject in this case being the defendant).[36] On examination the hypnotist in the case contended that the subject had very little conscious control and would therefore be unable to lie in response to questions asked by the hypnotist. He testified that the statements made by a person under hypnosis would, with "reasonable medical certainty," be truthful and correct. He further stated that, except in the case of certain mental disorders, the use of hypnosis would find the facts. In this case, the court allowed the hypnotist to ask questions whenever it appeared that the defendant was having difficulty understanding the attorney's questions. The procedure has been criticized as inherently suggestive.

CONCLUSION

To obtain an ideal climate for an effective psychiatric evaluation, a number of legal reforms would be necessary that might be unwise either from a social or legal point of view. If this is the case, then psychiatrists and jurists should realize the limitations that the legal procedure places on the accuracy and effectiveness of the psychiatric examination and, in turn, on the psychiatric opinion. But is psychiatry here being used more for its prestige value than for its probative value? And who is the reliable witness? Just thee and me, and I am not so sure about thee and thee is not so sure about me.

NOTES

1. An early and graphic illustration is provided by the *Song of Roland*—the duel between Thierry and Pinabel to decide the fate of Ganelon. See Stephenson, C. *Mediaeval Feudalism* 34. Ithaca, N.Y.: Cornell University Press, 1942.
2. Green, L. Jury Trial and Mr. Justice Black. *Yale L.J.* 65:482, 1965.
3. Goodhart, A. A Changing Approach to the Law of Evidence. *Va. L. Rev.* 51: 759, 761, 1965.
4. Rowley, S. The Competency of Witnesses. *Iowa L. Rev.* 24:482, 491–492, 1939.
5. Holdsworth, W. S. *History of English Law.* (3d ed.). London: Methuen, 1927.
6. It is unusual for a proposed witness today to be ruled incompetent and disqualified, except possibly in the case of the very young or the very old. That it does occur occasionally, however, is illustrated by the criminal case of *People v. McCaughan*, 49 Cal.2d 409, 317 P.2d 974 (1957), which involved the prosecution of a psychiatric aide at a state mental hospital charged with the involuntary manslaughter of one of the patients resulting from use of excessive force in spoon feeding. The patient, a 70-year-old woman, had refused to eat, believing that the food was poisoned. The prosecutor offered, as witnesses against the accused, other patients at the hospital. Perhaps seeking to protect the aide from criminal conviction, the California Supreme Court ruled that the court below had committed error because these witnesses had a history of insane delusions regarding the same matter as did the deceased. The decision is criticized in Note. *S. Cal. L. Rev.* 32:65, 1957. In another criminal case, *People v. Lapsley*, 26 Mich. App. 424, 182 N.W.2d 601 (1970), patients in a state mental home were allowed to testify against the defendant for torturing another patient, a 14-year-old girl. The witnesses, all minors with mental problems, were examined by the judge prior to their testimony and deemed to be mentally competent for testimonial purposes.
7. *Robertson v. Hackensack Trust Co.*, 1 N.J. 304, 317, 63 A.2d 515, 521 (1949) —concurring opinion.
8. The chapter titles in one book on cross-examination include: "Break Your Witness," "Step by Step Attack," "Witness on the Run," "The Kill," "Shock Treatment." Chapter titles of another book include "The Deposition Game," "Hold the Eye of the Witness," "Roll with the Punch," "Don't Beat a Dead Horse," "When Should Mud Be Thrown?", "Making Speeches While Objecting," "Endure the Torment," "Indirectly Depreciating the Witness," "How About Sarcasm?", "Hot on the Trial," "Stay in Command," "Don't Telegraph Your

Punch," "Preserve the Damaging Answer," "You Are Awfully Expensive, Doctor."

9. "Cross-examination elicits the truth in innumerable ways: by forcing the witness to abandon his prepared positions and improvise under circumstances of stress; by inducing the witness to elaborate his inventions; by striking down the inventions and leaving the witness exposed, so that the truth is his only available alternative. The resourceful techniques for dislodging a lie are as many as an agile mind can devise. Cross-examination is the only scalpel that can enter the hidden recesses of a man's mind and root out a fraudulent resolve. Psychiatry and drugs may have given us new insights into motivation, but the classic Anglo-Saxon method of cross-examination is still the best means of coping with deception, of dragging the truth out of a reluctant witness, and assuring the triumph of justice over venality." Nizer, L. *My Life in Court.*

10. Roucke, F. Psychological Research on Problems of Testimony. *J. Soc. Issues* 13:50, 1957.

11. Reversed in *Quercia v. United States,* 289 U.S. 466, 471-72 (1933). Consider also a recent hearing for alimony, where the husband said he paid $111 monthly on a loan. The wife's lawyer asked him what he did with the loan, and he replied that he spent the money on race horses and gambling. "That's an honest witness," remarked the judge. New Orleans *Times-Picayune,* Jan. 22, 1966, p. 1. Notwithstanding the self-destructive tendencies of people, the law considers that a damaging statement ("declaration against interest") has a circumstantial guarantee of trustworthiness. Jefferson, B. S. Declarations Against Interest: An Exception to the Hearsay Rule. *Harv. L. Rev.* 58:1, 1944; Morgan, E. Declarations Against Interest. *Vand. L. Rev.* 5:451, 1952. Pinocchio's nose increased in length whenever he told a fabrication. Benedetto Croce said, "The wood out of which Pinocchio is carved is humanity itself." The nose may be a symbolic displacement upward of the only human organ that varies in size depending on state of mind. The symbolic linkage can be traced to ancient times. Hollender, M. H. The Nose and Sex. *Med. Aspects Hum. Sexual.,* Dec. 1972, p. 84.

There is a growing literature on the proposition that people speak a nonverbal language with their bodies that can convey more about what they really mean than any words. See Bacon, A. M. *A Manual of Gestures.* Chicago: Burdett, 1893; Barnlund, D. C., and Haiman, F. S. *The Dynamics of Discussion.* Boston: Houghton Mifflin, 1960; Birdwhistell, R. L. *Kinesics and Context.* Philadelphia: University of Pennsylvania Press, 1970; Bruner, J. S., and Goodnow, J. J. *A Study of Thinking.* New York: Wiley, 1957; Cherry, C. *On Human Communication.* Cambridge: M.I.T. Press, 1961; Critchley, M. *The Language of Gesture.* London: Arnold, 1939; Davitz, J. R. *The Communication of Emotional Meaning.* New York: McGraw-Hill, 1964; Efron, D. *Gesture and Environment.* New York: King's Crown, 1941; Fast, J. *Body Language.* Philadelphia: Evans, 1970; Feldman, S. S. *Mannerisms of Speech and Gesture.* New York: International Universities Press, 1959; Fromm, E. *The Forgotten Language.* New York: Grove, 1951; Goffman, E. *Interaction Ritual.* New York: Anchor, 1967; Goffman, E. *The Presentation of Self in Everyday Life.* New York: Anchor, 1959; Hall, E. T. *Silent Language.* New York: Doubleday, 1959; Hall, E. T. *The Hidden Dimension.* New York: Doubleday, 1966; Hayakawa, S. I. *Language in Thought and Action.* New York: Harcourt, Brace, 1949; Jourard, S. M. *The Transparent Self.* New York: Van Nostrand, 1964; Jung, C. G. *Man and His Symbols.* New York: Doubleday, 1964; Maslow, A. H. *Motivation and Personality.* New York: Harper, 1954; Miller, G. H. *Language and Communication.* New York: McGraw-Hill, 1951; Morris, C. W. *Signs, Language and Behavior.* New York: Braziller, 1955; Morris, D. *Intimate Behaviour.* New York: Random House, 1971; Nierenberg, G. I. *How to Read a Person Like a Book.* New York: Hawthorn, 1971; Ogden, C. K., and Richards, I. A. *The Meaning of Meaning.* New York: Harcourt, Brace, 1958; Ruesch, J., and Kees, W. *Nonverbal Communication.* Berkeley: University of California Press, 1959; Sondel, B. *To Win with Words.* New York: Hawthorn, 1968; Spooner,

O. *How to Read Character*. Brattleboro, Vt.: Greene, 1965; Thayer, L. *Communication: Concepts and Prospectives*. Washington, D.C.: Spartan Books, 1967; Thienemann, T. T. *Symbolic Behavior*. New York: Washington Square Press, 1968; Tinbergen, N. *Social Behavior in Animals*. London: Methuen, 1953; Weinberg, H. L. *Levels of Knowing and Existence*. New York: Harper & Row, 1960; Wolff, W. *Expression of Personality*. New York: Harper, 1943. Marcel Marceau, the mime artist, is described as "the most naked artist in the world." "He can never hide behind the battlements of words." *New York Times*, April 21, 1973, p. 21.

12. Freud, S. Psycho-analysis and the Ascertaining of Truth in Courts of Law (1906). In *Collected Papers*. Vol. 2. Pp. 13–24, 1924.

13. Compare also Gandhi's observation: "You can wake up a man who is asleep, but if he is merely pretending to be asleep, your efforts will have no effect upon him."

14. Dr. Bernard Diamond interprets Freud's essay as saying that the use of psycho-analysis for the obtaining of legal evidence is of a highly experimental nature, that it should be utilized only in the spirit of research, and that the results should never be allowed to influence the verdict of the court. Diamond, B. Criminal Responsibility of the Mentally Ill. *Stan. L. Rev.* 14:59, 1961. That is not, however, my appreciation of Freud's essay.

15. In 1924, Colonel R. R. McCormick of the *Chicago Tribune* offered Freud $25,000, or anything he would name, to come to America to psychoanalyze Leopold and Loeb, presumably to demonstrate that they should not be executed. Hearing that Freud was ill, Hearst was prepared to charter a special liner so that Freud could travel undisturbed by other company. Freud declined both offers. Freud said, "I would say that I cannot be supposed to be prepared to provide an expert opinion about persons and a deed when I have only newspaper reports to go on and have no opportunity to make a personal examination." Jones, E. *The Life and Work of Sigmund Freud*. Vol. 1. London: Hogarth Press, 1953. This is an especially interesting observation in view of the controversial Bullitt-Freud book on Woodrow Wilson, recently published.

On another occasion, in a letter of November 4, 1920, from Vienna to Dr. Emil Oberholzer, Freud said: "My appearance as expert witness in the litigation concerning [not against] Wagner Jauregg didn't exactly mean the beginning of a new p[sycho]a[nalytic] era for Vienna. On the first day of the litigation, while I was present, the learned counsel behaved ever so sweetly. They used my absence the next day in order to bring out all the old, poisonous lies against p[sycho]a[nalysis]. I neither reacted myself, nor did I admit any reaction from another source. . . . ." (This letter is on file in the Menninger Museum, Topeka, Kansas.)

16. Munsterberg, H. *On the Witness Stand*. New York: Clark Boardman, 1923.

17. Wigmore, J. Professor Munsterberg and the Psychology of Testimony. *Ill. L. Rev.* 3:999, 1909.

18. *United States v. Hiss*, 88 F. Supp. 559 (S.D.N.Y. 1950).

19. *New York Times*, Jan. 6, 1950.

20. Correspondence of November 23, 1965, to Ralph Slovenko from Dr. Carl Binger, quoted with permission. See Hill, W. P. The Use and Abuse of Cross-examination in Relation to Expert Testimony: The Second Alger Hiss Trial. *Ohio St. L.J.* 15:458, 1954.

21. This phrase is used in the state's "Supplemental Memorandum" to *People v. Jones*, 42 Cal.2d 219, 266 P.2d 38 (1954), a pioneering case in which the court said that if the crime on charge involved a trait indicating a tendency toward sexual perversion, the accused may adduce expert psychiatric testimony that he is not a sexual deviate. The case is critically examined in Falknor, J. F. and Steffen, D. T. Evidence of Character: From the "Crucible of the Community" to the "Couch of the Psychiatrist." *U. Pa. L. Rev.* 102:980, 1954; but it is viewed with favor in Curran, W. Expert Psychiatric Evidence of Personality Traits. *U. Pa. L. Rev.* 103:999, 1955. A number of courts bar psychiatric testi-

mony of a witness's psychological condition. For example, in *Hopkins v. State*, 480 S.W.2d 212 (Tex. Crim. App. 1972), the defendant was convicted of unlawful possession of heroin largely on the testimony of a former heroin addict turned informer and undercover buyer for the police. Psychiatric testimony challenging the competence or credibility of the witness was not allowed. The court said that the divergence of psychiatric opinion and its frequent inexactness render its value minimal in enabling the jury to decide the issue of credibility. In fact, the court said, the jury after being subjected to several conflicting, equivocating and highly technical psychiatric opinions may actually be more confused than before. Another court said it failed to perceive the benefit to be gained from "an amateur's voyage on the fog-enshrouded sea of psychiatry." *United States v. Flores-Rodriguez*, 237 F.2d 405, 412 (2d Cir. 1956). See Note, *St. Mary's L. Rev.* 4:460, 1972.

22. Davidson, H.   Appraisal of the Witness, *Am. J. Psychiatry* 110:481, 1954. See also Dearman, H. B.   Psychiatric Examination of the Client. *Tenn. L. Rev.* 32: 592, 1965; Moore, E. H.   Elements of Error in Testimony. *Ore. L. Rev.* 28: 293, 1949. See generally Hoch, P. H., and Zubin, J. (Eds.).   *Psychopathology of Perception.* New York: Grune & Stratton, 1965; Smirnov, A. A.   *Problems of the Psychology of Memory.* New York: Plenum Press, 1973.
23. Davidson, *op. cit.*
24. Banay, R.   The Psychiatrist in Court. In Slovenko, R. (Ed.).   *Crime, Law and Corrections.* P. 433.
25. Comment, Psychiatric Evaluation of the Mentally Abnormal Witness. *Yale L.J.* 59:1324, 1950.
26. Monroe, R.   The Psychiatric Examination. In Slovenko, R. (Ed.).   *Crime, Law and Corrections.* P. 439.
27. 88 W. Va. 479, 107 S.E. 189 (1921).
28. In sex cases, utmost latitude in cross-examination of witnesses is usually permitted, because the accusation is easily made and difficult to disprove. The courts have permitted psychiatrists to expose mental defects, hysteria, and pathological lying in sex prosecutrices. See, e.g., *Mell v. State*, 133 Ark. 197, 202 S.W. 33 (1918); *People v. Rainford*, 58 Ill. App. 2d 312, 208 N.E. 2d 314 (1965); Note, *Syr. L. Rev.* 14:683, 1963. See also Blinder, M. G.   The Hysterical Personality. *Psychiatry* 29:227, 1966.
29. *State v. Concannon*, 25 Wash. 237, 65 Pac. 534, 537 (1901).
30. *State v. Fong Loon*, 29 Idaho 248, 158 Pac. 233, 236 (1916). The record in *Irwin v. Ashurst*, 158 Ore. 61, 74 P.2d 1127 (1938), discloses the following questions and answers:
Q. As much as I hate to I am going to have to ask you a personal question. Do you use narcotics?
A. No, sir, not now.
Q. You don't use any at all?
A. I was ill for ten years and the doctor gave me morphine at the time I had operations.
Q. You don't use them at all any more?
A. No.
During closing argument to the jury counsel said the following concerning the witness: "Did you watch her? Did you see how she acted? The mind of a dope fiend, she was full of it, she was full of it when she testified; she showed she was an addict; why, she's a lunatic, she's a crazy lunatic; she's a dope fiend; how nervous she was all through her testimony; she's a hop head; her whole testimony is imagination and delusion from taking dope; all through her testimony she showed it; she testified she had taken dope for ten years, and you may well know that she is still taking it; you know when a person has taken dope for ten years, they never stop it; she's a dope fiend; she is lower than a rattlesnake; a rattlesnake gives you warning before it strikes, but this woman gives no warning; she is under a delusion from taking narcotics as long as she has; on account of her being an addict, I wouldn't believe a word she said."

31. Comment, *Tul. L. Rev.* 34:389, 1960.
32. Zeligs, M. A. *Friendship and Fratricide—An Analysis of Whittaker Chambers and Alger Hiss.* Reviewed in Slovenko, R. *Int. J. Psychoanal.* 51:549, 1970.
33. 347 U.S. 556 (1954).
34. *State v. Butler,* 27 N.J. 560, 143 A.2d 530 (1958).
35. The Indiana Supreme Court and the California Court of Appeals have ruled that in sex-offender cases, when there is reason to doubt the truth of the accuser's allegations, a psychiatric examination should be made of the accuser to ascertain his or her mental and emotional condition and whether they have bearing on the accuser's credibility. The rulings stressed that the purpose of a psychiatric examination is "not to determine whether the witness is telling the truth, but to determine whether the emotional or mental condition of the witness may affect his or her ability to tell the truth." *Easterday v. Indiana,* 256 N.E.2d 901 (Ind. 1970); *California v. Francis,* 5 Cal. App. 3d 414, 85 Cal. Rptr. 61 (1970). However, in *Ballard v. Superior Court,* 64 Cal.2d 159, 49 Cal. Rptr. 302, 410 P.2d 838 (1966), a physician who was charged with the rape of a patient to whom he allegedly administered an intoxicating narcotic or anesthetic substance in order to prevent resistance could not obtain an order requiring the complaining witness to undergo a psychiatric examination for the purpose of determining whether her mental or emotional condition had affected her veracity. The trial judge rejected the request, under the power of discretion invested in him whether or not to order such an examination. A failure to order an examination is rarely held to be an abuse of discretion. See Juviler, M. Psychiatric Opinions as to Credibility of Witnesses: A Suggested Approach. *Calif. L. Rev.* 48:648, 1960.
36. *State v. Nebb,* No. 39540, Ohio C.P., Franklin Co., June 8, 1962; discussed in Note, Hypnosis in Court: A Memory Aid for Witnesses. *Ga. L. Rev.* 1:269, 1967.

4. Privileged Communication

A GENERAL principle of law is that the courts have a right to every man's evidence; but there are some justifiable exceptions, among them the privilege for certain confidential communications. Those covered by a testimonial privilege may withhold testimony or records notwithstanding a subpoena in any court proceedings as well as legislative and administrative proceedings.

The concept of privileged communication is based on the theory that the benefit to justice in allowing the testimony is outweighed by the injury to the relationship where the parties, fearing later disclosure, do not make full and adequate disclosure to one another. The argument for a psychotherapist-patient privilege essentially rests on the claim that it is the quality of the relationship between patient and therapist which is the catalyst for psychotherapeutic change.

The existence of a privilege would protect Freud's great invention of a unique human situation where a person, through a relationship with another, can explore the meaning and experiential realities of his life without intrusion. A basic assumption in psychotherapy is that a real relationship can be developed with the patient, one allowing the therapist and patient to work together profitably, only if there is no (collusive) contact or communication with others, including those who may have legal responsibility for the care of the patient. Everyone would agree that psychoanalytic psychotherapy cannot be conducted in a goldfish bowl.

A testimonial privilege, commonly known as a *shield law*, covers certain communications between specific classes of persons; thus, confessions made to ordinary people by friends are without any shield. The prevailing privileges cover the attorney-client, priest-penitent, physician-patient, and husband-wife relationships. In recent years legislatures have been requested to enact a privilege to protect confidential communications made to journalists, broadcasting and television newscasters, academic researchers, school teachers, social workers, marriage counselors, "confidential" clerks, accountants, stockbrokers, detectives, public officials, and trust companies. Privileges, however, are cautiously granted, after much hesitation, and then are narrowly interpreted because they lessen the evidence available to the court.

The history of the privilege covering psychiatrist-patient communication has its origins in the medical privilege which shields physician-patient communications. Being men of medicine, psychiatrists accordingly thought they should be subsumed under this medical privilege. Considering the social esteem of physicians, they thought that the medical privilege surely would be sacrosanct. There was, however, little justification for such a conclusion. Unknown in early common law, the privilege has been enacted in only about two-thirds of the states. The enactment originated at a time when contagious or infectious diseases were prevalent. Prior to the advances of medical science in combating disease, those plagued by the worst forms of infections (plague, leprosy, and venereal disorders) were practically isolated from society. The only means known to prevent the spread of contagion was to deny to the afflicted person all but the most limited forms of social intercourse; for example, the leper could not be a shopkeeper. A public statement that one had a contagious disease, as it tended to exclude him forever from the society of others, was considered highly defamatory; in a slander action, damage was "presumed and proof thereof unnecessary." To encourage medical visitation, New York in 1828 enacted the first medical confidential-communication privilege.

The seminal reason for the medical privilege long having disappeared, law commentators invariably have been critical of it. As a consequence, even where enacted, the privilege has been so strictly construed that there is apparently not one reported court decision in which the physician has been allowed to remain silent when subpoenaed to testify.

The National Conference of Commissioners on Uniform State Laws, which seeks to promote uniform legislation throughout the country, voted at its 1950 meeting that the physician-patient privilege should not be recognized. At the 1953 meeting, however, the Conference reversed its previous action and by a close vote decided to recommend the privilege as optional. The recommendation, however, contains so many exceptions that it is difficult to imagine a case in which it may be applied.

In every state, generally on the finding of waiver, the physician has been compelled to testify whenever his testimony has been relevant to the issues in the case. In the following situations exceptions to the privilege or waiver by the patient have been found necessary "in order to obtain information required by the public interest or to avoid fraud": communications not made for purposes of diagnosis and treatment; commitment and restoration proceedings; issues as to wills, or otherwise, between parties claiming by succession from the patient; action on insurance policies; medical reports required when treatment is rendered for venereal diseases, gunshot wounds, child abuse, etc.; communications made in furtherance of crime or fraud; mental or physical condition put in issue by the patient, as in personal injury cases; malpractice actions; and some or all criminal prosecutions (only Louisiana's privilege covers criminal cases). Thus, there is virtually nothing covered by the privilege. Rather than maintain a façade, the proposed *Federal Rules of Evidence*, governing the federal courts, omits the medical privilege. Nor is there a physician-patient privilege in the military; the *Manual for Courts-Martial* now specifically bars a privilege for psychotherapy.

Unlike the psychiatrist, the psychologist (or social worker) has no claim to coverage under the medical privilege unless he is working as an agent for a physician. In a number of states, however, including those without a medical privilege, the psychologists sought and obtained the enactment of a special psychologist-client privilege, often as part of the licensure or certification law. A few states likewise include a social-worker privilege in its statutes licensing the practice of social work. While most states do not provide a shield for information obtained by a social worker, a home visit, which statutes prescribe as condition for welfare assistance, does not fall within the Fourth Amendment's proscription against unreasonable searches and seizures. No state provides a research-subject or scholar's privilege.[1]

The Group for the Advancement of Psychiatry (GAP), in 1960, urged the enactment of special legislation to place psychiatrist-patient communications on the same basis as those between attorney and client.[2] When Professor Joseph Goldstein and Dr. Jay Katz of Yale University pointed out the difficulties which would arise from legislation by reference, GAP revised its proposal and urged the enactment of a long and detailed psychotherapist-patient privilege similar to that embodied in the Connecticut statute enacted in 1961.[3]

While the proposed *Federal Rules of Evidence* do not cover a physician who is asked about treatment of a purely physical ailment, they contain a psychotherapist-patient privilege, modeled in considerable measure on the Connecticut law. For the sake of uniformity, the federal enactment will likely influence other states to adopt a similar measure. Heretofore, the federal courts tended to follow the privilege law of the state in which it was sitting, although it was not compelled to do so.

The definition of *patient* is specifically spelled out as "a person who consults or is examined or interviewed by a psychotherapist for purposes of diagnosis or treatment of his mental or emotional condition"; the definition excludes persons submitting to examination for scientific purposes.

The definition of *psychotherapist* includes a medical doctor who devotes all or part of his time to the practice of psychiatry, and a licensed or certified psychologist who devotes all or part of his time to the practice of clinical psychology. It includes pretenders who are reasonably believed by their patients to be medical doctors, as well as general practitioners doing part-time counseling whether or not they have special qualifications. Unlicensed therapists and counselors of all kinds, however, including psychologists, can be required in court to reveal the confidences of those whom they have counseled, even if the patients thought what they were saying was privileged and believed the therapists to be licensed. The Advisory Committee says that the distinction made between unlicensed persons thought to be medical doctors and unlicensed persons doing psychotherapy "is believed to be justified by the number of persons, other than psychiatrists, purporting to render psychotherapeutic aid and the variety of their theories." It also appears that each participant in group therapy, under direction of one who is a psychiatrist or a licensed or certified psychologist, could assert the privilege to prevent any other member from testifying to what has been said in the group.[4]

The exceptions to the privilege contained in the Connecticut enactment and the new federal rule differ substantially from those of the attorney-client privilege because of the basic differences in the relationships. Rejecting the argument that the nature of a psychotherapist-patient relationship demands complete security against legally coerced disclosure in all circumstances, the committee of psychiatrists and lawyers who drafted the Connecticut statute concluded that in three instances—the areas where the privilege would most often have been claimed—the need for disclosure was sufficiently great to justify the risk of possible impairment of the relationship. These three exceptions are incorporated into the federal rule and are so broad that, like the recommendation in 1953 of the National Conference of Commissioners on Uniform State Laws, it is difficult to imagine a case in which the privilege applies.

In one exception, involving proceedings for hospitalization, it is said that the interests of both patient and public call for a departure from confidentiality. Since disclosure is authorized only when the psychotherapist determines that hospitalization is needed, control over disclosure is placed largely in the hands of a person in whom the patient has already manifested confidence, hence damage to the relationship is deemed unlikely. In a second exception, involving a court-order examination where the relationship is likely to be one entered into at arm's length, the exception is effective only with respect to the particular purpose for which the examination is ordered. Thus, for example, no statement made by the accused in the course of an examination into competency to stand trial is admissible on the issue of guilt. In a third exception, involving the patient's condition as an element of claim or defense, the patient, in fairness and to avoid abuses, is said to waive the privilege by injecting his condition into litigation. Similar conditions are said to prevail after the patient's death.[5]

Some six states currently have laws specifically granting special protection to the psychiatric relationship over and above that given to medical communications generally. In addition to the exceptions provided in the federal rule, some psychotherapist-patient-privilege statutes, enacted in some states, have an exception for child-custody cases (federal courts do not handle child-custody cases). For example, the Massachusetts law, enacted in 1968, denies the privilege "in any child-custody case in which either party raises the mental condition of the other party." Psychiatric testimony is made available here in an effort to provide for the best interests of the child.

California's psychotherapist-patient privilege, enacted in 1965, was recently tested in a much publicized case involving Dr. Joseph Lifschutz.[6] The proceedings arose out of a suit instituted by Joseph F. Housek, a high-school teacher, who brought a $175,000 damage suit against John Arabian, a student, for damages resulting from an alleged assault. Housek's complaint alleged that the assault caused him "physical injuries, pain, suffering, and severe mental and emotional distress." During the course of a deposition, Housek stated that he had received psychiatric treatment from Dr. Lifschutz over a six-month period approximately ten years earlier. The defendant then subpoenaed Dr. Lifschutz and all his medical records relating to the treatment of Housek. Dr. Lifschutz refused to produce any of his medical records and declined even to disclose whether or not Housek had consulted him or had been his patient.

Upon the psychiatrist's refusal to cooperate, defendant Arabian sought a court order compelling the production of the subpoenaed records and answers to questions on deposition. Relying on the patient-litigant exception, the court determined that because the plaintiff, in instituting the pending litigation, had put in issue his mental and emotional condition, the statutory psychotherapist-patient privilege did not apply. The privilege belongs to the patient, not to the physician, and is waivable by the patient. While the therapist may claim the privilege on behalf of his patient or ex-patient, if there is proof that the patient wants the communication made public, the therapist must comply. The privilege is a shield and may not be used as a sword, hence it is considered dissolved or waived by the patient when he makes a legal issue of his physical or mental condition.[7]

Statements made by a patient to a physician or psychiatrist as to the symptoms and effects of his injury or malady are admissible in evidence on his behalf, as an exception to the hearsay rule. Under the sporting theory of justice, it is only fair that the defendant have the benefit of the statements when they are favorable to him. Thus, when plaintiff Housek claimed that he had suffered "emotional distress" as a result of the injuries he had suffered, the privileged status of his communications with his psychiatrist was waived.

The permissible scope of the inquiry depends upon the nature of the injuries which the plaintiff-litigant himself has brought before the court. Disclosure is compelled only with respect to the mental condition put in issue; disclosure is not compelled with respect to other aspects of the patient-litigant's personality. Thus, in *Lifschutz*, for example, the defendant would not be authorized to demand plaintiff's psychotherapeutic communications be examined to determine if he has ever exhibited aggressive tendencies or other such personal attributes. The plaintiff had not put in issue such elements of his mental condition merely by instituting an action for damages resulting from assault.

If the issue in *Lifschutz*, however, had been "who started the affray?" rather than "did the damages result from the assault?" then evidence of character, i.e., whether or not the patient had ever exhibited aggressive tendencies, would have been relevant. The logic would be: "Quarrelsome men are more likely than others to commit assaults. Mr. X is quarrelsome; Mr. Y is peaceable. In an affray between the two, it is more likely that Mr. X was the aggressor."

In some situations the patient's pleadings may clearly demonstrate that his entire mental condition is being placed in issue and that records of past psychotherapy will be relevant. This is illustrated in a case where a mental patient in a prison hospital sought release, contending that he was not a dangerous or violent individual, as the state mental health officials asserted. When the patient's medical records were offered to substantiate the state's position, he claimed such records were privileged. The court, analogizing the facts before it to those of the patient-litigant exception to the medical privilege, found that "petitioner himself caused his mental condition to be put in issue by his application for habeas corpus and averments of his brief."[8]

The burden rests upon the patient initially to show that a given confidential communication is not directly related to the issue he has tendered to the court. This is because only the patient knows both the nature of the illness for which recovery is sought and the general content of the psychotherapeutic communications. The patient may have to delimit his claimed "mental or emotional distress" or explain, in general terms, the object of the psychotherapy in order to illustrate that it is not reasonably probable that the psychotherapeutic communications sought are directly relevant to the mental condition that he has placed in issue.

As the foregoing would suggest, the statutory privilege is just "much sound and fury signifying nothing." The practice in states where there is no physician-patient privilege or psychotherapist-patient privilege is the same as in states where there is a privilege. Moreover, in states which have enacted a privilege, the practice is found to be the same thereafter as it was before the enactment of the privilege.

The real test is one of relevancy, which arises regarding all evidence in every trial. In effect, this test, not privilege, governs the right of nondisclosure. The concept brings to mind the current student demand for relevance, or what has been called the glorification of the happening. Relevant evidence in law is "evidence having any tendency to make the existence of any fact that is of consequence to the determination of the action more probable or less probable than it would be without the evidence." In other words, does the item of evidence tend to prove that precise subject which is sought to be proved? In every case, where the testimony or records of a physician or psychotherapist have been required, it was because the evidence was deemed relevant to an issue in the case. As a consequence, in the last analysis, the confidentiality of a physician-patient or psychotherapist-patient communication is protected from disclosure only by showing that the communication would have no relevance to the issues in the case.

A priest-penitent communication may be relevant to an issue in a case, but the disclosure is nonetheless not demanded because of the deference given by the community to the relationship. Even in jurisdictions where there is no statutory priest-penitent privilege, an attorney would hardly dare subpoena a priest to testify regarding communications made by a penitent. It would not set right with judge or jury. It is not the enactment of a statutory privilege, but rather the feeling in the community about the relationship that makes a relationship sacrosanct. Likewise, an attorney rarely, if ever, subpoenas a secretary, even though the boss-secretary relationship is not protected by a statutory privilege, for the relationship is considered sacrosanct. (The word *secretary* is from Latin *secretum,* secret.) The physician-patient or psychotherapist-patient relationship is not considered untouchable by the community and therefore does not stand on the same footing as the priest-penitent or secretary-boss relationship.[9]

In many cases where a psychiatrist is subpoenaed, his testimony is not awaited with baited breath. The subpoena often has as its main purpose not investigation but rather intimidation of the patient into foregoing or settling the case. The privilege, at best, covers only the content of a communication and not the fact of a relationship; hence under a discovery demand, the identity of a treating psychiatrist can be elicited and then pressure can be brought to bear which frightens the patient into thinking that all his statements made in psychotherapy will be revealed in open court. In the nature of things, it is difficult to estimate the number of cases in which patients have dropped suits or feared to initiate them because of the apprehension of disclosure.[10]

A priest, who would not even be called to establish the fact of a relationship, is still very much considered a deputy of and answerable only to God. At one time the physician was considered in the same light. During the last century, however, as in the case of the sovereign king, the physician is no longer regarded as deriving his power from God. Nonetheless, for a long time the physician continued to be regarded with reverence because of the close relationship which he had with his patients. More recently, as personal-injury litigation multiplied, there have been demands made upon the physician for medical information regarding the litigant. At the same time, the physician-patient relationship has come to be regarded as a financial relationship and nothing more. Although the physician-patient relationship, as a result of lobbying, has been buttressed by statutes providing a communication privilege, the courts drew into them an exception when the patient put his health into issue; the result of this exception, apart from others, for all practical purposes was to dissolve the privilege.

In his argument against the medical privilege, the leading commentator on the law of evidence, Wigmore—who was not an enthusiastic advocate of testimonial privilege generally—maintained that a communication of a patient to a physician rarely originates in a confidence that it will not be disclosed. The idea that confidence is intended, which is the basis of the Hippocratic oath, often seems contrary to the reality of a situation. Except when afflicted with syphilis and other loathsome diseases, the patient seeks out opportunities to discuss his ailment with family, friends, neighbors and, in fact, with anyone who will listen. People often injure themselves or develop symptoms for the purpose of gaining attention and affection. Wigmore wrote: "In only a few instances, out of the thousands daily occurring, is the fact communicated to a physician confidential in any real sense. From asthma to broken ribs, from ague to tetanus, the facts of the disease are not only disclosable without shame but are in fact often publicly known and knowable by everyone except the appointed investigators of the truth."[11] The same argument is sometimes now made to undercut the psychotherapist privilege, namely, that people speak publicly in great detail about their psychiatric sessions. This argument, however, overlooks the fundamental fact that the individual's sense that it is he who decides when to "go public" is a crucial aspect of his feeling of autonomy.

To deal with the situation, a number of psychiatrists have said that they will refuse to testify, although required by law to do so, and will risk a jail term or a fine or both. In a well-publicized case some years ago, Dr. Roy Grinker, when called upon to testify about a patient in therapy, said on the stand, "I cannot answer in good conscience." Although Illinois at the time had no statutory privilege and his testimony would have been relevant to the case, he was not cited for contempt. Perhaps it was the judge's disposition toward psychiatry or Dr. Grinker's stature as a psychiatrist that kept him out of contempt.[12]

Attorneys recognize that attempts to gouge testimony out of a psychiatrist on the witness stand may result in distorted or perjured statements, so they may resort to a subpoena of records. To protect records, some psychiatrists and hospitals are keeping two sets, one for the law in the case of subpoena and the other for treatment. The concealment or destruction of records is a flagrant violation of the law and is not to be condoned.

Rather than manipulate the law by the keeping of double records, it is advised that the best protection that can be ensured the patient is the exercise of extreme caution in writing records. Some psychiatrists keep no records at all, although records might provide protection to the psychiatrist in the event of suit against him by the patient for malpractice in treatment. Dr. Marc Hollender at one time said:

> I do not keep any records at all. Very candidly, I do not want any records that could ever be subpoenaed into court and records cannot be subpoenaed if they do not exist. I do not keep records other than the form cards that my secretary makes out, listing the dates of appointments and my charges and collections, and that's it.
>
> I did keep records some years with the idea that I was collecting pure gold, that some day I would refine into Journal articles. Then one day I

woke up and came to the conclusion that this was nonsense. I did not have a precious metal. At best I had a few alloys and what I really wanted to write was probably in my head anyway. So at that point I had a big bonfire, and since that day I have not written anything other than brief notes about things that I especially wanted for some purpose quite detached from the patient.[13]

Dr. Gregory Zilboorg years earlier suggested that psychiatrists make no notes, in order to assure confidentiality. It is an echo of a practice followed generally by people in some other countries: "Don't keep papers —rely on your memory."

The privilege's exceptions, for all practical purposes, render the privilege a nullity. As a shield, it provides very little protection. Aside from no record keeping, one solution is that the psychiatrist also be a priest, for then he could, like a character in William P. Blatty's book, *The Exorcist*, say, "I can always tell the judge it was a matter of confession."

NOTES

1. As the medical or psychotherapist privilege covers the treatment situation, and not research, the psychiatrist or other professional person engaged in social- or behavioral-science research would not be covered by it. Scientists and investigators ask for a researcher's or scholar's testimonial privilege, contending that freedom of scholarship to investigate without fear to the investigated is of paramount importance. (Query as to who would qualify as a researcher or scholar under the proposal.) A. C. Kinsey, concerned with obtaining the confidence of his subjects, developed elaborate techniques, including the development of a code with the guidance of an experienced cryptographer. He stated: "If we were brought before a court we would have to hope that such precedents would be extended to scientists involved in the investigation of such a subject as human sex behavior. If the courts of all levels were to refuse to recognize such a privilege, there would be no alternative but to destroy our complete body of records and accept the consequences of such defiance of the courts. If law enforcement officials, students of law, and persons interested in social problems want scientific assistance in understanding such problems, they will have to recognize a scientist's right to maintain the absolute confidence of his records, for without that it would be impossible to persuade persons to contribute to this sort of study." Pomeroy says: "There is no question that Kinsey would have gone to any lengths to prevent disclosure, as he vowed. We were prepared to destroy the records and throw ourselves on the mercy of the court." Pomeroy, W. B. *Dr. Kinsey and the Institute for Sex Research.* New York: Harper & Row, 1972. Arthur L. Liman, general counsel to the New York State Special Commission on Attica, reportedly also said he would destroy the records of the confidential interviews he held with prison inmates, or even go to jail, before he would turn them over to anyone outside the commission. The state prosecutor preparing criminal cases stemming from the prison uprising had subpoenaed the records of 3,000 confidential interviews conducted by the commission. *New York Times,* Sept. 13, 1972, p. 34. See generally Butler, R. N. Privileged Communication and Confidentiality in Research. *Arch. Gen. Psychiatry* 8:139, 1963; Nejelski, P., and Lerman, L. M. A Researcher-Subject Testimonial Privilege: What to Do Before the Subpoena Arrives. *Wis. L. Rev.* 1971:1085; Ruebhausen, O. M., and Brim, O. G. Privacy and Behavioral Research. *Colum. L. Rev.* 65:1184, 1965; Notes, *J.A.B.A.* 58:520, 868, 1972;

Harvard Professor Jailed in Pentagon Papers Case. *New York Times*, Nov. 22, 1972, p. 1.
2. Group for the Advancement of Psychiatry: Report No. 45. *Confidentiality and Privileged Communication in the Practice of Psychiatry*, June 1960.
3. Goldstein, J., and Katz, J. Psychotherapist-Patient: The GAP Proposal and the Connecticut Statute. *Am. J. Psychiatry* 118:733, 1962. Goldstein and Katz were members of the committee that prepared the Connecticut bill.
4. Rule 504 of the proposed *Federal Rules of Evidence*, providing a psychotherapist-patient privilege, states:

(*a*) *Definitions.*
(1) A "patient" is a person who consults or is examined or interviewed by a psychotherapist for purposes of diagnosis or treatment of his mental or emotional condition.
(2) A "psychotherapist" is (i) a person authorized to practice medicine in any state or nation, who devotes all or a part of his time to the practice of psychiatry, or is reasonably believed by the patient so to be, or (ii) a person licensed or certified as a psychologist under the laws of any state or nation, who devotes all or a part of his time to the practice of clinical psychology.
(3) A communication is "confidential" if not intended to be disclosed to third persons other than those present to further the interest of the patient in the consultation, examination, or interview, or persons reasonably necessary for the transmission of the communication, or persons who are participating in the diagnosis and treatment under the direction of the psychotherapist, including members of the patient's family.
(*b*) *General Rule of Privilege.* A patient has a privilege to refuse to disclose and to prevent any other person from disclosing confidential communications, made for the purposes of diagnosis or treatment of his mental or emotional condition, among himself, his psychotherapist, or persons who are participating in the diagnosis or treatment under the direction of the psychotherapist, including members of the patient's family.
(*c*) *Who May Claim the Privilege.* The privilege may be claimed by the patient, by his guardian or conservator, or by the personal representative of a deceased patient. The person who was the psychotherapist may claim the privilege but only on behalf of the patient. His authority so to do is presumed in the absence of evidence to the contrary.
(*d*) *Exceptions.*
(1) Proceedings for Hospitalization. There is no privilege under this rule for communications relevant to an issue in proceedings to hospitalize the patient for mental illness, if the psychotherapist in the course of diagnosis or treatment has determined that the patient is in need of hospitalization.
(2) Examination by Order of Judge. If the judge orders an examination of the mental or emotional condition of the patient, communications made in the course thereof are not privileged under this rule with respect to the particular purpose for which the examination is ordered unless the judge orders otherwise.
(3) Condition an Element of Claim or Defense. There is no privilege under this rule as to communications relevant to an issue of the mental or emotional condition of the patient in any proceeding in which he relies upon the condition as an element of his claim or defense, or, after the patient's death, in any proceeding in which any party relies upon the condition as an element of his claim or defense.

The rule is a provision of the new code of evidence for all federal courts, the first ever drafted, and is based largely on a seven-year study by a committee of the United States Judicial Conference, the administrative agency of the federal court system. The proposed rules have eleven basic sections and 76 rules with a multitude of sub-sections. The eleven sections are entitled: *General Provisions; Judicial Notice; Presumptions; Relevancy and Its Limits; Privileges; Witnesses;*

Opinions and Expert Testimony; Hearsay; Authentication and Identification; Contents of Writings, Recordings, and Photographs; and *Miscellaneous Rules.* The existing rules of evidence in federal courts are the product of separate developments in each of the 93 federal districts over the years. Although the new rules will not eliminate the authority of individual federal judges in their own courtrooms to adjust the rules to particular cases (such decision seldom reversed on appeal), the rules afford much greater uniformity, and would tend to discourage forum shopping. The general thrust of the new rules is to permit the use of more kinds of evidence and to discard many old restrictions on admissibility. Symposium on the Proposed Federal Rules of Evidence. *Wayne L. Rev.* 15:1061; 16:135, 1969.

The rules were scheduled to go into effect July 1, 1973, unless vetoed by the Congress. The rules, however, evoked considerable criticism. A number of the provisions were attacked as substantive. The authority of the court to formulate rules of evidence which partake more of substance than procedure is subject to controversy. *New York Times,* Feb. 1, 1973, p. 9; Feb. 4, 1973, p. 10-E; Feb. 8, 1973, p. 13; Feb. 9, 1973, p. 16. Shortly after their submission, Congress on March 19, 1973, delayed the effective date of the rules and required affirmative congressional approval before they become effective. Adoption of the rules is expected in calendar year 1973, but in any event, it is anticipated that state courts will take a close look at some or all of the rules with a view to adoption for their own proceedings. Brinton, H. T. The Proposed Federal Rules of Evidence: Pointing the Way to Needed Changes in Illinois. *John Marshall J. of Prac. & Proc.* 5:242, 1972.

One of the controversial elements in the area of privilege, other than the newspaperman's claim for privilege, was instigated by Dr. Ernest B. Howard, Executive Vice-President of the American Medical Association. In essence, he wrote to the chairmen of both judiciary committees decrying the absence of physician-patient privilege. He saw Rule 504 as a replacement for the old physician-patient privilege. As a result, he advocated the deletion of Rule 504 and reintroduction of the proposed physician-patient privilege found in the 1953 Uniform Rules of Evidence, although this rule, as carried out in various states, is so full of deductions that it offered no shield whatsoever to any patient communication. Then again, as pointed out in this chapter, Rule 504 likewise offers a pierceable shield. History has a way of repeating itself.

5. Advisory Committee's Notes. *Federal Rules of Evidence.*
6. *In re Lifschutz,* 2 Cal.3d 415, 467 P.2d 557, 85 Cal. Rptr. 829 (1970). The *Lifschutz* case was featured on the Law page of *Time,* April 1970, p. 60, and was also reported at numerous meetings of psychiatric societies and in psychiatric and psychoanalytic bulletins and newsletters. To cover legal expenses the Northern California Psychiatric Society made a nationwide appeal to psychiatrists for contributions. The American Psychoanalytic Association and the National Association for Mental Health filed amicus curiae briefs.
7. Another example of waiver is found in a recent New York case where a former mental patient claimed damages for mental and psychological problems resulting from an accident following his release. He had been in the mental hospital four years prior to the accident. The defendant sought to inspect the records of the mental hospital. The court held that when the plaintiff claimed that the accident was the cause of his mental condition, he placed his mental condition in issue and therefore waived the statutory privilege of confidentiality granted him under the provision of state law. [*Mancinelli v. Texas Eastern Transmission Corp.,* 308 N.Y.S.2d 882, 33 N.Y. App. 105 (1970).] See also Annot., 44 A.L.R.3d 797.

In an action by a doctor's widow and children for his wrongful death in a shooting incident, testimony by the treating psychiatrists of both the wife and the deceased doctor (who had been undergoing psychoanalysis) tending to show the doctor's state of mind, his belief of his wife's infidelity, his mental turmoil, his intention to terminate the marriage and support, and his entire attitude toward his wife and children was relevant to the damage issue and hence was admissible. [*Allen v. Riedel*, 425 S.W.2d 665 (Tex. Civ. App. 1968).] Illinois recently enacted an amendment to the patient-litigant exception, which provides that *both* patient and psychiatrist have privilege in divorce cases even though "mental cruelty" is the ground for divorce, unless either the patient or psychiatrist introduces testimony concerning communications between them. Beigler, J. S. The 1971 Amendment of the Illinois Statute on Confidentiality: A New Development in Privilege Law. *Am. J. Psychiatry* 129:311, 1972.

An independent psychiatric examination for the purposes of a possible trial has been held not to give immunity to the treatment situation. In a recent California case, the plaintiff, a young girl, who sought damages for emotional trauma allegedly resulting from an automobile collision, stated in the course of a deposition that prior to the collision she had had no problems necessitating psychiatric care but thereafter she had felt the need because she blamed herself for the accident in which her mother and brother were killed. The testimony and records of the psychiatrist were thereupon sought. The psychiatrist claimed that disclosure would be harmful to the patient, because a betrayal of confidence would affect her treatment. He stated that the need for therapy had arisen either wholly or partially from the accident; but he contended that an independent psychiatric evaluation by another psychiatrist, which had been done, could determine the specific effects of the collision on the plaintiff and would be more useful than his records. The effect of any disclosure by him, he urged, could prevent the continuation of therapy and might "conceivably result in even more catastrophic things like a suicide attempt." The court, however, ruled that there is no privilege as to a communication relevant to an issue concerning mental or emotional condition tendered by the patient. [*Murphy v. Hall*, Calif. Court of Appeal, Oct. 19, 1971; *Psychiatr. News*, Feb. 2, May 17, 1972, p. 1.] See also *Psychiatr. News*, March 7, 1973, p. 1.

In support of the decision, psychiatrist Samuel D. Lipton observed: "Who [is] able to provide better evidence: the psychiatrist who examined her immediately after the accident and continued to treat her, or one who saw her for the first time much later? If one assumes that the court has the obligation to demand the best evidence available, then it is disingenuous to equate the two sources. The issue that confronts the court is not secrecy but the claimant's demand for money. No one has forced her to initiate her suit, and if that secrecy is vital, all she need do is abandon it. On the other hand, the court neither wants, needs, nor will it even permit the disclosure of irrelevant evidence or the exposure of a litigant to humiliation. The question is whether the claimant should be entitled both to get the money and, in addition, to shroud what might be the best source of evidence in total secrecy." [Letter, *Psychiatr. News*, March 15, 1972, p. 2.] In response, psychiatrist Jerome S. Beigler says: "[The claim] that 'the court will not permit the disclosure of irrelevant evidence or the exposure of a litigant to humiliation' . . . is simply not true. There have been too many instances in which the opposite was true." [Letter, *Psychiatr. News*, May 3, 1972, p. 2.] See also Letters, *Psychiatr. News*, May 17, 1972, p. 2.

In Michigan, the privilege is deemed waived only if the plaintiff brings an action to recover for personal injuries or for malpractice *and* if the plaintiff shall produce in his own behalf any physician as a witness who has treated him for such injury. [*Eberle v. Savon Food Stores*, 30 Mich. App. 496, 186 N.W.2d 837 (1971).] Some courts have held that an allegation of pain and suffering does not ipso facto place mental condition in issue as an element of a personal-injury claim. [*Tylitzki v. Triple X Service*, 126 Ill. App.2d 144, 261 N.E.2d 533 (1970).]

8. *In re Cathey*, 55 Cal.2d 679, 12 Cal. Rptr. 762, 361 P.2d 426 (1961).
9. A rare court appearance of a clergyman occurred in *Wirtanen v. Prudential Ins. Co.*, 27 Mich. App. 260, 183 N.W.2d 456 (1970), involving a claim against an insurance company for recovery under a double indemnity clause. The defendant-insurer claimed that the deceased had committed suicide by shooting himself with a shotgun; the plaintiff claimed it was an accident. To support its conten-

tion, the defendant called to the stand a minister who testified that he had talked to the deceased before he died. The defendant asked the minister whether or not the deceased had told him how the mortal injury occurred. The witness was allowed to answer "yes" but no further inquiries were permitted on the basis of the priest-penitent privilege. The court of appeals held that it was error to allow even the preliminary question and answer. A rare appearance of a stenographer occurred in *Wolfle v. United States*, 291 U.S. 7 (1934), where the testimony of the stenographer, reading from her notes the content of a letter dictated by a husband to his wife, was used against him. The husband-wife marital privilege was not applicable in the case because "husband and wife may conveniently communicate without stenographic aid"; the stenographer was deemed a third-party whose presence polluted confidentiality. [Note, *Wash. & Lee L. Rev.* 9:91, 1952.] In any event, the case does not represent an intrusion upon the secretary-employer relationship since the communication was intended for transmittal to others.

10. In the attorney-client relationship, the identity of the attorney's client will seldom be a matter communicated in confidence, for the procedure of litigation ordinarily presupposes a disclosure of that fact. Every litigant is entitled to know the identity of his opponent. While the considerations are different, it is also said that a patient's identity is not protected from disclosure under the medical or psychotherapist privilege. [Note, *Texas L. Rev.* 39:512, 1960.]

11. Wigmore, J. *Treatise on System of Evidence in Trials at Common Law.* Vol. 8. Boston: Little, Brown, 1961. §§2380, 2380(a).

12. *Binder v. Ruvell*, Civil Docket 52C2535, Circuit Court of Cook County, Illinois, June 24, 1952; reported in *JAMA* 150:1241, 1952, and discussed in *Nw. U.L. Rev.* 47:384, 1952.

13. Discussion at Annual Meeting, May 1963, at Section on Private Practice of the American Psychiatric Association, in program on "The Medico-Legal Aspects of Private Psychiatric Practice," published in *J. Dis. Nerv. Syst.* 26:169, 1965.

II. THE PSYCHIATRIST AND EVALUATION IN CRIMINAL LAW

5. CRIMINAL RESPONSIBILITY

THE interplay of law and psychiatry has found most expression in the topic of criminal responsibility. The consequence of this focus has been to make it the conceptual center of law-psychiatry. The annual Isaac Ray award lectures, begun in 1952 under the auspices of the American Psychiatric Association, have dealt mainly with criminal responsibility. The recent murder trials of John L. Frazier, Charles Manson, Jack Ruby, Richard Speck, and Sirhan Sirhan have again spotlighted the function and significance of the plea "not guilty by reason of insanity," which at times has made the psychiatrist himself and his theories seem frivolous.

Full sanctions for deviations from standards of conduct, which might be called "the rules of the game," are not applied when there is a valid excuse. In ordinary affairs a child who vomits on another is not punished for it, since the vomiting was an involuntary act and not his fault. An offender who claims insanity asks to be treated in effect as if he were an infant at the time of the act. In common parlance, the formula of excuse is, "I couldn't help it" or "I didn't know what I was doing." A statement from a doctor is often required as a voucher. This sense of justice pervades the law; thus, one who urinates on the street violating an ordinance may get a doctor's note that he has bladder trouble.

Evidence of insanity relates to the issue of intent. Any proposal to abolish the insanity defense, which has been urged from time to time, makes no vital change in the law as long as intent or a certain state of mind is a required element of crime. With moral guilt an essential ingredient of the criminal law, testimony in one form or another about the accused's state of mind would continue.

For centuries, it has been considered unjust to label a person as criminal or blameworthy unless his unlawful act was performed with a guilty mind (*mens rea*). In the place of an eye for an eye, tooth for tooth, the Greeks allowed an excuse, the first time, in the case of Orestes, who was "driven" to kill his mother in order to avenge his father. Reduced states of competency vary in terms of their power to excuse. Sleepwalking may absolve an individual. On the other hand, drunkenness, on occasion, can increase the fault instead of diminishing it.

The law on criminal intent, as Justice Holmes once said, takes account of incapacities only when the weakness is marked, such as "infancy and madness." Otherwise expressed, one is held accountable in criminal law only when he is "competent to commit crime." The formulation of the rule theoretically determines the function of the court, the function of the jury, the instructions of the judge to the jury, and the scope of the evidence. Various tests have been formulated to determine when a person is sufficiently demented or defective as not to be held accountable for his acts.

Today, criminal responsibility is determined in England and in the majority of jurisdictions in the United States according to the rule formulated in 1843 following the trial in England of a Scotsman by the name of Daniel M'Naughten. In this well-known case, M'Naughten (a paranoid schizophrenic, if labeled today) felt persecuted by the Tories, who were then in power. He decided to take action against them by killing Sir Robert Peel, the prime minister. He kept a watch on Peel's house, and when he saw a man come out, he shot Edward Drummond in the mistaken belief that he was shooting Peel. The jury, as instructed, found the defendant not guilty on the ground of insanity. The acquittal was the beginning rather than the end of this celebrated case.[1]

Although acquitted of crime, M'Naughten was certified as being of unsound mind and detained in a lunatic asylum, where he spent his remaining 22 years. The verdict of not guilty on the ground of insanity, however, created a furor, and within a few days after the trial the case was debated in the House of Lords. It was speculated that M'Naughten, a Scotsman, was a political assassin. The times were turbulent. Shortly before, Queen Victoria had been the target of an attempted assassination by an assailant who was also found not guilty by reason of insanity. On learning of the M'Naughten acquittal, she summoned the House of Lords to an extraordinary session. They were instructed to clarify and tighten the concept of criminal responsibility. They came forth with the so-called M'Naughten rules. These rules are extensive, but the pronouncement of greatest import provides:

> The jurors ought to be told in all cases that every man is presumed to be sane and to possess a sufficient degree of reason to be responsible for his crimes, until the contrary can be proved to their satisfaction; and that, to establish a defence on the ground of insanity, it must be clearly proved, that, at the time of the committing of the act, the party accused was labouring under such a defect of reason, from disease of the mind, as not to know the nature and quality of the act he was doing or, if he did know it, that he did not know he was doing what was wrong.

M'Naughten himself probably would not have been exculpated under the legal definition of insanity laid down in the test that bears his name. In a literal application of the M'Naughten rule, two (and probably only two) classes of lawbreakers would be exempted from punishment: for example, in the case of homicide: (1) the person thought that the gun with which he shot somebody was not a deadly weapon but a water pistol and was therefore unaware of the fact that it would kill (he did not "know the nature and quality of the act he was doing"); or (2) a person labored under the delusion that he was physically attacked and acted in legitimate self-defense ("he did not know he was doing what was wrong"). The question to be asked under the M'Naughten rule is not whether the lawbreaker knew the difference between right and wrong in general. Rather the question is whether in the particular matter he "knew he was doing what was wrong," that is, whether he was under such a delusion that he thought he acted in legitimate self-defense.

The M'Naughten rule has been criticized mainly because it concerns itself with cognition or intellectual understanding and makes no reference to emotion. A person, although not laboring under a defect of reason, may be incapable of controlling his behavior. The judges formulating the M'Naughten rule were aware that crime, like all human conduct, has multiple etiology, but they decided upon a narrow exculpatory provision. Under the M'Naughten rule as formulated, a person is not exempted from criminal responsibility because his choice of action is determined or affected by pathology. He is exempted when he lacks moral judgment.

Adherence today to the old M'Naughten rule of 1843 may be taken to signify any of the following: (1) the M'Naughten rule as formulated is a dead horse and is only given lip service; (2) psychiatry and law have not progressed during the past 130 years; (3) no change or improvement is needed in the law; or (4) criminal responsibility under the M'Naughten rule involves a moral issue, unaffected by developments and knowledge in the field of psychiatry.

Today, the M'Naughten rule is given lip service. Psychiatric testimony has been freely admitted in establishing "disease of the mind" and in interpreting the word *know* in the phrase "know he was doing what was wrong." *To know* includes more than simply knowledge that something is wrong; it includes, the courts say, a reasonably adequate grasp of the implications of the act.

Notwithstanding the broad scope being given the M'Naughten rule, Judge Bazelon of the Court of Appeals for the District of Columbia in 1954 in *Durham v. United States* ruled that the trial had not been adequate because the expert witness had not been permitted to present his full testimony. In the place of the M'Naughten rule, Judge Bazelon, looking at the New Hampshire law, formulated a "disease-defect-product" test which provides:

> An accused is not criminally responsible if his unlawful act was the product of mental disease or mental defect.[2]

The Durham decision expressly states that the purpose of the rule is to open the inquiry to the widest possible scope of medical or psychiatric testimony. It sought to remove the shackles, although theoretical, of the M'Naughten rule; it sought to call a spade a spade. In formulating his opinion, Judge Bazelon relied heavily on the advice of leading forensic psychiatrists.

The decision was widely heralded. Dr. Karl Menninger at the time described it as "more revolutionary in its total effect than the Supreme Court decision regarding segregation." Forensic psychiatrists Lawrence Z. Freedman, Manfred Guttmacher, and Winfred Overholser together published a statement recommending its wide adoption, saying, "The Durham decision permits free communication of psychiatric information." Dr. Gregory Zilboorg called it "a step toward enlightened justice." The American Psychiatric Association awarded Judge Bazelon a certificate of commendation proclaiming that "he has removed massive barriers between the psychiatric and legal professions and opened pathways wherein together they may search for better ways of reconciling human values with social safety."

As it turned out, however, the Durham rule has resulted in confusion and a plethora of appeals. In cases where the rule has been employed, judges and jurors alike have been mired in confusion over the terms *disease*, *defect*, and *product*. With the exception of Maine, and a modification of it in New Mexico, the rule did not spread beyond the District of Columbia.

In 1961, after a few years of the rule's application, Judge Bazelon's colleague in the District of Columbia—Judge Burger, now Supreme Court Chief Justice—angrily stated: "Not being judicially defined, these terms (*mental disease* or *defect*) mean in any given case whatever the expert witnesses say they mean. We know also that psychiatrists are in disagreement on what is a 'mental disease,' and even whether there exists such a definable and classifiable condition. . . . [N]o rule of law can possibly be sound or workable which is dependent upon the terms of another discipline whose members are in profound disagreement about what those terms mean."[3]

The sweeping use of the terms *mental disease* or *defect* was only part of the problem. The product test brought in all the controversies of psychic determinism versus free will. What does *product* mean? Is every criminal act related to mental disorder? Is anyone accountable for his acts? Judge Holtzoff, district judge in the District of Columbia, observed: "It is not inconceivable that perhaps the so-called Durham formula would not have been adopted if it had been foreseen at the time that it would lead to the exculpation of sociopaths or psychopaths from criminal liability."[4]

Judge Bazelon, too, became disillusioned; in 1964, he said, "The frequent failure to adequately explain and support expert psychiatric opinion threatens the administration of the insanity defense in the District of Columbia."[5] In 1967, in an apparent act of desperation, Judge Bazelon took the unusual step of writing the following set of instructions, to accompany all orders requiring mental examinations, advising psychiatric witnesses as to how they should function:

Dr. _____, this instruction is being given you in advance of your testimony as an expert witness, in order to avoid confusion or misunderstanding. The instruction is not only for your guidance, but also for the guidance of counsel and the jury.

Because you have qualified as an expert witness your testimony is governed by special rules. Under ordinary rules, witnesses are allowed to testify about what they have seen and heard, but are not always allowed to express opinions and conclusions based on these observations. Due to your training and experience, you are allowed to draw conclusions and give opinions in the area of your special qualifications. However, you may not state conclusions or opinions as an expert unless you also tell the jury what investigations, observations, reasoning, and medical theory led to your opinion.

As an expert witness, you may, if you wish and if you feel you can, give your opinion about whether the defendant suffered from a mental disease or defect. You may then explain how defendant's disease or defect relates to his alleged offense, that is, how the development, adaptation, and functioning of defendant's behavioral processes may have influenced his conduct. This explanation should be so complete that the jury will have a basis for an informed judgment on whether the alleged crime was a "product" of his mental disease or defect. But it will not be necessary for you to express an opinion on whether the alleged crime was a "product" of a mental disease or defect and you will not be asked to do so.

It must be emphasized that you are to give your expert diagnosis of the defendant's mental condition. This word of caution is especially important if you give an opinion as to whether or not the defendant suffered from a "mental disease or defect" because the clinical diagnostic meaning of this term may be different from its legal meaning. You should not be concerned with its legal meaning. Neither should you consider whether you think this defendant should be found guilty or responsible for the alleged crime. These are questions for the court and jury. Further, there are considerations which may be relevant in other proceedings or in other contexts which are not relevant here; for example, how the defendant's condition might change, or whether he needs treatment, or is treatable, or dangerous, or whether there are adequate hospital facilities, or whether commitment would be best for him, or best for society. What is desired in this case is the kind of opinion you would give to a family which brought one [o]f its members to your clinic and asked for your diagnosis of his mental condition and a description of how his condition would be likely to influence his conduct. Insofar as counsel's questions permit, you should testify in this manner.

When you are asked questions which fall within the scope of your special training and experience, you may answer them if you feel competent to do so; otherwise you should not answer them. If the answer depends upon knowledge and experience generally possessed by ordinary citizens, for example questions of morality as distinguished from medical knowledge, you should not answer. You should try to separate expert medical judgments from what we may call "lay judgments." If you cannot make a separation and if you do answer the question nonetheless, you should state clearly that your answer is not based solely upon your special knowledge. It would be misleading for the jury to think that your testimony is based on your special knowledge concerning the nature and diagnosis of mental conditions if in fact it is not.

In order that the jury may understand exactly what you mean, you should try to explain things in simple language. Avoid technical terms whenever possible. Where medical terms are useful or unavoidable, make sure you explain these terms clearly. If possible, the explanation should not be merely general or abstract but should be related to this defendant, his behavior and his condition. Where words or phrases used by counsel are unclear, or may have more than one meaning, you should ask for clarification before answering. You should then explain your answer so that your understanding of the question is clear. You need not give "yes or no" answers. In this way any confusion may be cleared up before the questioning goes on.

Some final words of caution. Because we have an adversary system, counsel may deem it is his duty to attack your testimony. You should not construe this as an attack upon your integrity. More specifically, counsel may try to undermine your opinions as lacking certainty or adequate basis. We recognize that an opinion may be merely a balance of probabilities and that we cannot demand absolute certainty. Thus you may testify to opinions that are within the zone of reasonable medical certainty. The crucial point is that the jury should know how your opinion may be affected by limitations of time or facilities in the examination of this defendant or by limitations in present psychiatric knowledge. The underlying facts you have obtained may be so scanty or the state of professional knowledge so unsure that you cannot fairly venture any opinion. If so, you should not hesitate to say so. And, again, if you do give an opinion, you should explain what you did to obtain the underlying facts, what these facts are, how they led to the opinion, and what, if any, are the uncertainties in the opinion.[6]

Not too optimistic about the instruction, Judge Bazelon in a footnote made the "following observations for himself": "It may be that this instruction will not significantly improve the adjudication of criminal responsibility. Then we may be forced to consider an absolute prohibition on the use of conclusory legal labels. Or it may be that psychiatry and the other social and behavioral sciences cannot provide sufficient data relevant to a determination of criminal responsibility no matter what our rules of evidence are. If so, we may be forced to eliminate the insanity defense altogether or refashion it in a way which is not tied so tightly to the medical model. . . . But at least we will be able to make that decision on the basis of an informed experience."[7]

Having once expressed great optimism about the possibilities of the Durham decision, Menninger in his 1968 book, *The Crime of Punishment,* recanted: "We psychiatrists should keep out of the courtroom. We don't belong there. We cannot function effectively there. It is not our proper sphere of action. We do not understand the language addressed to us nor convey what we intend to and think we do, using the language we employ. Our performance in the courtroom ritual is a continuation of what is really a fraudulent, discriminatory, undemocratic procedure—that of trying to manipulate psychiatric categories and legal sanctions for the special benefit of selected individuals. And the Durham decision doesn't help matters—in spite of our hopes."[8]

Disheartened by both the M'Naughten and Durham rules, Judge Biggs of the Court of Appeals for the Third Circuit (which has jurisdiction over federal cases in Delaware, New Jersey, Pennsylvania, and the Virgin Islands) in 1961 drew from the test proposed by the American Law Institute (ALI) in its *Model Penal Code* in deciding *United States v. Currens.* The incapacity-for-self-control test set out in *Currens* is that criminal responsibility will not be imposed upon one who was suffering from a disease of the mind and did not possess substantial capacity to conform his conduct to the requirements of the law at the time for the criminal act.[9]

The ALI's *Model Penal Code,* prepared during the years 1952 to 1962, recommends a combination of the right-wrong test and an updated version of irresistible impulse:

(1) A person is not responsible for criminal conduct if at the time of such conduct as a result of mental disease or defect he lacks substantial capacity either to appreciate the criminality (wrongfulness) of his conduct or to conform his conduct to the requirements of the law; (2) As used in this article, the terms "mental disease or defect" do not include an abnormality manifested only by repeated criminal or otherwise antisocial conduct.

A number of states that operate under the M'Naughten rule have extended the ground of the insanity plea through an addition known as *irresistible impulse.* The defendant may have known what he was doing and known that it was wrong, but nevertheless may have been unable to resist an overwhelming impulse to commit the crime. This test is included in subsection (1) of the ALI standard. The test when originally formulated in 1897 read: "Though conscious of [the nature of the act he is committing] and able to distinguish between right and wrong and know that the act is wrong, yet his will [that is,] the governing power of his mind, has been otherwise so completely destroyed that his actions are not subject to it, but are beyond his control." The formulation in subsection (2) of the ALI standard is designed specifically to include persons diagnosed as of psychopath or antisocial personality within the scope of criminal responsibility.

Then, in 1972, eighteen years after its adoption of the Durham rule, the Court of Appeals for the District of Columbia took the occasion in *United States v. Brawner* to discard it. In this case, the court had ordered the American Psychiatric Association, American Psychological Association, American Civil Liberties Union, National District Attorneys Association, National Legal Aid and Defender Association, and the Georgetown Legal Intern Project to submit briefs as amici curiae on such issues as the adoption of the ALI test for criminal responsibility and the possibility of the complete abolition of the insanity defense. The case was argued twice.

In its amicus curiae brief, the American Psychiatric Association suggested the rejection of the Durham test and endorsed instead the ALI standard. The amicus brief further suggested that if the court were to reject the ALI test, then the abolition of the insanity defense would be an alternative acceptable to the psychiatric profession. It stated that it would favor, with appropriate safeguards, abolishing the insanity defense, but it recognized that the abolition of the defense would have to be accomplished by constitutional amendment.[10]

The court, all nine members sitting *en banc*, including Judge Bazelon, unanimously decided in a 143-page opinion to throw out its Durham rule and adopt in its place the ALI standard. In a year of deliberation of the case, the court considered and rejected the alternatives of abolishing the insanity defense entirely or of adopting a standard allowing the jury to decide sanity based simply on the question of whether the accused "can justly be held responsible." The court said that it rejected the abolition of the insanity defense because such an action should come from the legislative branch of government, not the judicial. (The Supreme Court on a number of occasions has indicated that where an insanity defense is raised, the failure to afford a defendant a fair and impartial hearing on the question is a denial of due process of law.) It said that it rejected allowing juries to decide sanity based on their own judgment because such a procedure "would place too heavy a burden on the jury." In general, the court reasoned that the Durham rule did not work because of the latitude it gives expert witnesses to make value judgments in front of the jury. The "value judgments" referred to come in the form of medical or psychiatric testimony.

The ALI test of criminal responsibility is rapidly being accepted throughout the country. Of the eleven federal jurisdictions, all but one (the First Circuit, which has jurisdiction over federal cases in Maine, Massachusetts, and New Hampshire) now use it. The Currens test of the Third Circuit eliminates the phrase "either to appreciate the criminality of his conduct or," and adds to the phrase "requirements of law" the words "which he is alleged to have violated." In addition, the ALI standard is now used in some nine states (Idaho, Illinois, Indiana, Kentucky, Massachusetts, Missouri, New York, Vermont, Wisconsin).

The *irresistible impulse* concept raises the difficult question: how can you differentiate between an impulse that was truly irresistible and one that simply was not resisted? In its application, the psychiatric expert is invariably asked the policeman-at-the-elbow question on cross-examination. "Would the defendant have committed this act if a policeman were standing next to him at the time?" An effective answer may be, "Your guess is as good as mine." Jack Ruby fatally shot Lee Harvey Oswald before a television audience right inside Dallas police headquarters. There is less likelihood that a defense of irresistible impulse will stand up when there is evidence of premeditation and planning as they tend to demonstrate well-reasoned behavior or reasoned intent.

No matter which test of criminal responsibility is applied, the psychiatrist's testimony must describe the offender's state of mind at the time of the commission of the offense. It is necessary to project back from the time of examination to the time of the offense. The validity of an opinion on the defendant's mental condition at some given moment in the past—weeks or months prior to the examination—is invariably challenged on cross-examination. Information obtained from acquaintances and those who had custody of the defendant (jailers) following the crime is helpful.

In arriving at his opinion, the expert is expected to have made or have had carried out the full battery of psychological tests (Rorschach, Thematic Apperception Test, Bender Gestalt, Minnesota Multiphasic Personality Inventory), and physiological tests (x-ray examination, physical examination, electroencephalogram, and neurological examination). Failure to apprise oneself of certain facts or test results or failure to use available examination techniques makes the expert vulnerable for the question, "Would that change your opinion, doctor?" Another attack on adequacy of examination involves questioning the amount of time that the expert spent with the accused.

Flight from the scene, attempts to avoid detection, and the circumstances of the apprehension of the accused are all relevant to the psychiatric examination. If the defendant after the crime said that he was sorry that he did it or showed regret or remorse, the prosecutor may argue that this is an indication that he knew he had committed a wrongful act. In one case, the prosecutor proceeded this way in cross-examining the defense psychiatrist:

Q. So I ask you, sir, in your opinion . . . was he or did he indicate in any way that he was sorry that he killed this girl?
A. He did not say he was sorry he had killed this girl and he was expecting the electric chair.
Q. Doctor, can't you answer that question Yes or No?
A. I can only answer it on the basis of what I observed. I observed that . . .
Q. What is your opinion, doctor? Was he or was he not sorry that he killed the girl?
A. My opinion was that he regretted killing the girl but somehow felt it was in the cards, that something like this was going to happen in his life, and that he had no control over it, and this is the way it was going to be, he was going to get the chair and here it comes.
Q. So your answer is, doctor, that in your opinion from your examination of him he was sorry that he killed the girl. That is true, isn't it?
A. I would say he was sorry but felt there was nothing he could do about it.
Q. Doctor, are you trying to hedge on the answer?
A. I am trying to give you an accurate answer as to what I felt was going on in this man's mind.

In the various tests of criminal responsibility as well as in other areas of the law, the rule on competency is grounded on an old demon-possession theory. In early times, disease or physical illness (e.g., a heart attack) was considered to come from the outside, and this was also the explanation given for mental disorder. The insane were regarded as possessed by demons, and they were dealt with accordingly ("the Devil was beat out of them"). The Talmud says: "No man commits a crime except when a spirit of madness is entered into him." In the New Testament, Matthew (17:15–18) tells of Jesus curing a "lunatick" by rebuking a devil which departed from him that very hour. A sneeze has been thought to blow evil spirits out of the body. "God bless you" is said when someone sneezes. By the ninth or tenth century, psychological problems had become fully enmeshed with those of theology. The terms *devil's sickness* and *witch disease* became more and more used. As late as the sixteenth century, Ambroise Paré, the father of modern surgery, believed that the devil caused women to become witches and that witches should be destroyed. Strangely, however, in some periods of time certain disorders—epileptic seizures and hallucinations—were considered to be sent by the gods as tokens of special grace, and the afflicted persons were revered. In the days of George III, last king of the English colonists in what is now the United States, the two houses of Parliament passed a bill authorizing the court physicians to scourge the lunatic king. Psychiatrists today look for the "underlying disorder."

Although the criminal-law tests do not mention demons, mental illness, as used in these tests, is regarded essentially as a form of demoniacal manipulation. Under the M'Naughten, Durham, or ALI rule, it is necessary to establish a disease or defect of the mind. Under the M'Naughten test, it is not sufficient simply to show that the accused did not know that what he was doing was wrong—"disease of the mind" must be the cause. Under both Durham and ALI tests, the crime or incapacity for self-control must be the product of a "mental disease or defect."

The concept pervades other areas of the law. The test on competency to stand trial requires that the accused's inability to understand the proceedings or assist counsel must be the product of a mental disease or defect. Civil commitment law provides for the hospitalization of a person who is mentally ill and who, as a consequence, is dangerous to himself or others, or is in need of care or treatment. Also, in the test on competency to make a will, the testator's inability to understand the nature and extent of his property and the objects of his bounty must be the result of a mental disease or defect. Only in the area of tort law is there no search for mental disease or mental defect.[11]

Mental disorder, apart from organic lesions such as a syphilitic infection of the brain, has no locus. The expansive way in which the concept is used, though, is an example of the error which A. N. Whitehead called *misplaced concreteness*, that is, an abstraction is taken to be a concrete entity. It is the result of reification, the need to make a thing out of a process. In this case the process that is made into a thing is a way or style of life.

When the defense of insanity is raised in criminal cases, much ritual is adhered to, but how do juries actually decide whether the accused is legally insane? Attempting to answer this question, Rita James Simon in *The Jury and the Defense of Insanity* reports on a controlled experiment, introducing three variations into the record.[12] The first variation was designed to test whether it makes any difference which criteria of mental incapacity—M'Naughten, Durham, or neither—a court directs the jury to apply. It was found that a jury instructed under the M'Naughten test is more likely to convict than is a jury instructed under Durham; whereas an uninstructed jury is likely to return the same verdict as a Durham jury. The second variation in the record was designed to test the effect were the jury to hear a considerably more elaborate evaluation of the accused's illness than is ordinarily given by psychiatrists in a case involving mental incapacity. No difference in the verdicts was found. The third variation was designed to determine whether verdicts would vary when there was an instruction that a verdict of not guilty on grounds of mental incapacity would necessarily result in commitment of the accused to a psychiatric hospital. Again, the variation was found to result in no difference. This result is not surprising, in light of the fact that over 90 percent of the jurors assumed, without being told, that an automatic commitment procedure was in force. Judges in many states instruct the jury on the consequences of their verdict.

If and when an accused is found insane, he is exculpated, but nonetheless, his freedom is curtailed. He has been shown to be either a person who does not know what he is doing or one who cannot control his conduct which has resulted in serious harm to another. In the same manner as did the House of Lords following the M'Naughten decision, Congress and the various states have enacted legislation providing for commitment of any person who is acquitted on grounds of insanity. Commitment is made to a unit for the criminally insane, subject to release only upon a judicial finding that he "has recovered his sanity and will not in the reasonable future be dangerous to himself or others." Regarding the entire procedure, Menninger aptly says: "Millions of dollars are spent annually to determine who has [responsibility] or hasn't it. If one is found to have it, he is locked up; if he is found not to have it, he is also locked up."[13]

From the considerable (mostly critical) discussion surrounding the insanity defense, it would appear that it is invoked or prevails in every criminal case although, in fact, its use or success is rare. It is estimated that only 2 percent of homicide cases lead to acquittal by reason of insanity. In a turgid essay, penned about 1870, Mark Twain ridiculed the insanity defense, saying that rank criminal offenders were resorting to its use to escape the reach of the law, and he called for a law against the practice. The essay is entitled, *A New Crime—Legislation Needed*, the *new crime* being the use of the insanity defense. Mark Twain was perhaps unaware that the procedure was a device to temper the use of the death penalty, and unlike the jurors recently polled by Simon, he also presumed that these offenders were released. He apparently was not mindful of the fact that offenders acquitted on the plea of insanity are confined in a criminally insane unit of a mental hospital or penal institution. They do not walk out of the courthouse, free men.

It was for that reason that on the suggestion of the prosecution, the jury in the trial of James Hadfield in 1800 returned what was, at that time, a novel verdict: "We find the prisoner is Not Guilty; he being under the influence of insanity at the time the act was committed." He was detained for the rest of his forty years. Under the Insanity Bill of 1800, the court was empowered to order persons acquitted on account of insanity to be kept in strict custody, "in such place and such manner as the court may decide, during the King's pleasure."

The insanity defense at one time was frequently urged. The severity of punishment for felonies—usually death—begat in practice certain loopholes in no way related to the merits of the case. During the recent past, with the steady demise of the death penalty, and even of life imprisonment, the insanity defense has been less frequently raised or entertained, usually only when other defenses such as alibi or self-defense were unavailing.[14] It is preferable to be sent to the criminal unit of a mental hospital (with the possibility of release) than to be executed; but when the choice is between prison or a criminally insane unit, the option is for prison. The prison is a more comfortable facility than the criminally insane unit, and the term of confinement is fixed, and usually for a shorter period of time.

An analysis of data gathered on the actual administration of the defense of insanity and competency to stand trial, which is discussed in the next chapter, was recently conducted under the auspices of the American Bar Foundation.[15] It yielded these findings:

1. From a practical point of view the importance of the defense of insanity has been greatly exaggerated in the professional literature, in the public mind, and in the law itself. Criminal responsibility cases constitute a small percentage of all cases; defendants, given the alternatives, choose not to plead insanity as a defense because of the plea's drawbacks, stemming both from its procedural difficulties and from the consequences of success.

2. Psychiatric testimony is not excluded or seriously fettered under the M'Naughten right-wrong test of responsibility.

3. The procedure for inquiry into competency to stand trial is the critical phrase in the classification and disposition of mentally disturbed criminal defendants.

4. The competency referral in some localities has become the vehicle for a medically oriented pretrial screening of defendants accused of misdemeanors and minor felonies. In practice the competency-to-stand trial concept is manipulated to achieve one or another objective, and the inquiry procedure tends to become submerged in questions of appropriate disposition, dangerousness, commitability, and treatment.

5. The alternative of civil commitment is widely employed for disposition of minor offenders, as is outpatient psychiatric care when it can be provided.

6. At all stages of operation, there is a severe shortage of psychiatric resources. The scarcity of mental health resources produces difficulties in every phase of the criminal law's administration.

7. There is poor communication and much conflict of purpose between agencies sharing responsibility for disposition of mentally disturbed offenders. Little cooperation is discernible between the different agencies administering criminal justice and the medical agencies with which they deal. Each agency is preoccupied with its own immediate concerns.

When facts of the commission of the offense are undeniable—consider, for example, Jack Ruby's slaying of Lee Harvey Oswald or Arthur Bremer's shooting of Governor George Wallace—the defense of insanity, a subjective element, is the only tactic that a defense attorney has available to furnish judge or jury so that they may exercise discretion in the case. Hence, a defense attorney is obliged to argue the apparently fanciful, as was argued in the Bremer case, "This kid is pure schizophrenic . . . the kid's old lady is to blame for his mental disorders."

The administration of the law is not a mechanical operation; it needs avenues for the exercise of discretion. The insanity plea is an excuse for behavior, the policy question being the extent to which an excuse will be tolerated.[16] In law-school courses on criminal law and procedure, emphasis is on rights of suspects and not on rights of victims. Individuals apparently tend to identify more with the offender than with the offended. It may be said that the law on criminal responsibility stems out of our fear of being accused or held accountable for something we may have done or imagined, even though beyond our reason or control. St. Augustine expressed thanks that he was not responsible for his dreams, which caused him embarrassment.

NOTES

1. *Daniel M'Naughten's Case*, 10 Clark & Fin. 200, 8 Eng. Rep. 718 (1843). There is no agreement on the spelling of the defendant's name. It is variously spelled M'Naghten, M'Naughton, McNaughten, and McNaughton. The original report of the trial spelled it M'Naughton. The most common spelling—M'Naghten —is probably the least correct. A photograph of his signature seems to read, Mc-

Naughtun, which prompted Justice Frankfurter to ask, "To what extent is a lunatic's spelling of his own name to be deemed an authority?" Diamond, B. L. On the Spelling of Daniel M'Naghten's Name. *Ohio S.L.J.* 25:84, 1964.

2. *Durham v. United States*, 214 F.2d 862 (D.C. Cir. 1954).
3. *Blocker v. United States*, 288 F.2d 853, at 859, 860 (D.C. Cir. 1961).
4. *O'Beirne v. Overholser*, 193 F. Supp. 652, at 660 (D.C. 1961).
5. *Rollerson v. United States*, 343 F.2d 269, at 271 (D.C. Cir. 1964).
6. Appendix, *Washington v. United States*, 390 F.2d 444, at 457 (D.C. Cir. 1967).
7. 390 F.2d at 457.
8. See Menninger, K. *The Crime of Punishment.*
9. 290 F.2d 751 (3d Cir. 1961). Professor Joseph Goldstein of the Yale Law School recently suggested at a meeting of the American Psychoanalytic Association that people who are caught up in a riot may be regarded as lacking the capacity to control their behavior, for the individual who is lost in the anonymity of a crowd bent on mischief may be said to have lost any normal ability to hold his impulses in check. Consider gang rape, discussed in Geis, G. Group Sexual Assaults. *Med. Aspects Hum. Sexual.*, May 1971, p. 101.
10. *United States v. Brawner*, 471 F.2d 969 (D.C. Cir. 1972); noted in *N.Y.U. L. Rev.* 47:962, 1972.
11. *McGuire v. Almy*, 297 Mass. 323, 8 N.E.2d 760 (1937).
12. Simon, R. J. *The Jury and the Defense of Insanity.* Reviewed in Wise, E. M. Book Review. *N.Y.U. L. Rev.* 43:603, 1968.
13. Menninger, K. *The Human Mind* (3d ed.). Pp. 7–8. Demonology is discussed in Greeley, A. M. The Devil, You Say. *New York Times Magazine*, Feb. 4, 1973, p. 15; Lurie, A. Witches and Fairies. *N.Y. Review of Books*, Dec. 2, 1971, p. 6; Stone, L. The Disenchantment of the World. *N.Y. Review of Books*, Dec. 2, 1971, p. 17. See also Dalman, C. J. Criminal Behavior as a Pathologic Ego Defense. *Arch. Crim. Psychodynam.* 1:555, 1955; Roche, P. Q. Criminality and Mental Illness—Two Faces of the Same Coin. *U. Chi. L. Rev.* 22:324, 1955.
14. The insanity defense raised to a charge of willful failure to file an income tax return, for example, is rarely considered to have merit, as might be expected. [*United States v. Baird*, 414 F.2d 700 (2d Cir. 1969).] In one case upholding the conviction of an attorney who claimed that mental strain caused him to neglect his own tax affairs, the Tax Court said, "He clearly knew he owed tax, knew he was required to file returns, and knew he had done neither." See *Wall Street J.*, Oct. 18, 1972, p. 1. In one state property tax case, though, it was ruled that that there was sufficient evidence to hold that an 83-year-old plaintiff, seeking recovery of his property, was unable to understand the nature and effect of his failure to pay back taxes or the fact that such failure would result in a loss of his property. [*Dayiantis v. Blackhawk, Inc.*, 189 N.W.2d 808 (Mich. App. 1971).]
15. Matthews, A. R. *Mental Disability and the Criminal Law.* Chicago: American Bar Foundation, 1970.
16. See Austin, J. A Plea for Excuses. In *Philosophical Papers.* Oxford: Oxford University Press, 1961. Chap. 6, p. 123; Hart, H. L. A. The Ascription of Responsibility and Rights. In Flew, A. G. N. (Ed.). *Logic and Language.* Oxford: Blackwell, 1955. Chap. 8, p. 145. See also Scott, M. B., and Lyman, S. M. Accounts. *Am. Soc. Rev.* 22:46, 1968.

6. COMPETENCY TO STAND TRIAL

THE law on competency to stand trial relates to fairness. An altruistic concept, it provides that a person accused of crime may be placed on trial only if he is able to understand the nature of the charge against him and aid counsel in preparing his defense. The rule is an aspect of the general prohibition against trials in absentia. The individual who fails to meet the test may be physically present in the courtroom but, in the vernacular, is out of it mentally.

According to the Supreme Court, it is not enough that the trial judge find "the defendant is oriented to time and place and has some recollection of events," but the "test must be whether he has sufficient present ability to consult with his lawyer with a reasonable degree of rational understanding—and whether he has a rational as well as factual understanding of the proceedings against him."[1] Paradoxically, the defense attorney, who best knows whether or not the client is able to cooperate with him, is not the only party who may raise the issue of the defendant's competency to stand trial. Instead, in many jurisdictions, the prosecutor often invokes the plea, as he did in the cited case which went to the Supreme Court.

The rule on competency to stand trial originated in cases of physical disability. Thus, if the accused had a heart attack or appendicitis, his trial would be postponed until such time as he would be physically able to be present. The notion developed subsequently that a person so disoriented or removed from reality that he could not properly participate and aid in a meaningful defense ought not to be put to trial. Simply put, the rule says, "A case is to be put off until the accused is able to stand trial." It provides for a continuance of the trial. As frequently happens, however, rules take on new purpose in the process of application. The rule, by and large, has been turned into a form of putting away undesirables for an indefinite time.

QUERIES REGARDING COMPETENCY

The law on competency to stand trial raises several queries: (1) Is mental illness or insanity an essential component to incompetency to stand trial? (2) What is the usual interpretation of triability held by a psychiatrist? (3) Is it appropriate for a psychiatrist to respond to a literal application of the test? (4) Does the actual operation of the test correspond to its literal interpretation? (5) What is the effect of the so-called courtroom decorum cases on the test? (6) Is it possible to get along without the test?

Is Mental Illness an Essential Component?

William of Occam in the early fourteenth century recommended that concepts or entities not be multiplied unnecessarily. The concept is known as *Occam's razor*. One might wonder whether the mental-illness or insanity concept adds anything to the competency test. Does not the term *insanity* here mean merely inability to understand the charges and to assist counsel? A purely operational procedure would ask simply whether the person understands the charges and can assist counsel.

It is usually said, however, as in other tests of competency, that the incompetency must be "the result or product of mental disease or defect," and the psychiatrist is called upon to testify to the existence of that disease or defect. A mental disease or defect is thus made a necessary but not sufficient condition. It must be the cause of the enumerated effects. The *Model Penal Code* states, "No person who *as a result of mental disease or defect* lacks capacity to understand the proceedings against him or assist in his own defense shall be tried, convicted, or sentenced for the commission of an offense as long as such incapacity endures" (emphasis added).

What Is the Usual Interpretation of Triability Held by a Psychiatrist?

A prediction of the accused's ability to perform is made at a competency hearing where the psychiatrist is invariably called upon for his appraisal. Often the psychiatrist is under the impression that he is governed by the much publicized M'Naughten rule of criminal responsibility, the time-of-offense or substantive rule on guilt or innocence. At a competency hearing, counsel may clarify the rule for the expert, but even at that time it is often not done, and at times there may be no opportunity because psychiatric reports are frequently submitted by mail to the court.

The M'Naughten rule is so well publicized that it is not surprising that it is thought to pervade all spheres of the law. Indeed, some psychiatrists have even used the M'Naughten rule in assessing a testator's competency to make a will. In law, unlike in psychiatry or medicine, a term is context-defined, depending on the legal issue. Thus, the term *insanity* is variously defined in law to test, for example, capacity to commit crime, to stand trial, or to make a will.[2]

*Is It Appropriate for a Psychiatrist to Respond to a Literal
Application of the Test?*

Apart from the psychiatrist's appreciation of the legal test on triability, a literal application of the test also raises the question of whether or not he is the appropriate person to respond, even though his recommendation is advisory only. The psychiatrist has no special knowledge of what is required to understand criminal charges or to assist counsel. One would assume that the matter would be best left to the accused's own counsel.[3]

To be sure, if the defendant's counsel seeks to stay or postpone trial by claiming that his client is incapable of standing trial, the claim can and should be verified, since it is also in the interest of the state to have a speedy trial. In general, police investigation or surveillance of the accused is the best way to detect malingering. Psychiatric experts are surely not needed to investigate this claim. The original intent of the test was to excuse only flagrantly psychotic and defective individuals. An unsophisticated layman or the custodial officer is able to apply the test; only a commonsense point of view is needed for a literal application of the test. There would appear to be no need for a diagnosis in depth and certainly not for Rorschach protocols. The sort of evaluation needed for measuring triability is not the same as that needed for psychiatric treatment.

Rudolf Hess, Hitler's deputy as Nazi Party leader, was brought to the Nuremberg trials from England (whereto he had mysteriously fled in 1941) in an apparent state of total amnesia. Among his belongings were small packages of food which he had reportedly wrapped, sealed, and labeled during a period of paranoid delusions concerning food poisoning. Captain G. M. Gilbert, prison psychologist at the Nuremberg trials, reports in his *Nuremberg Diary* that Hess sat in his cell all day in a state of apathetic absentmindedness, having not the slightest inkling of familiarity with any subject from his past. When confronted by Hermann Goering and Franz von Papen, he failed to recognize either of them. "There was little doubt in our minds," says Gilbert, "that he was essentially in a state of complete amnesia."

A few days before the beginning of the trial, Hess was examined in his cell by an American psychiatric commission consisting of Dr. Nolan D. C. Lewis of Columbia University, Dr. Donald E. Cameron of McGill University, and Colonel Paul Schroeder of Chicago. Continuous questioning gave no indication that Hess's amnesia was anything but genuine although the psychiatrists concluded that he was not legally insane. Hess's defense counsel argued to the court that Hess was not competent to defend himself because of his amnesia, while the prosecution argued that he was competent to defend himself since the psychiatrists had found him not insane. After about an hour and a half of such argument, Hess surprised the court by declaring, "My memory is again in order. The reasons why I simulated loss of memory were tactical. In fact, it is only my capacity for concentration that is slightly reduced. . . . Hitherto in conversation with my defense counsel I have maintained my loss of memory. He was, therefore, acting in good faith when he asserted that I lost my memory."

The court adjourned in pandemonium. Goering was at first incredulous but then roared with delight at what he took to be Hess's joke on the court and the psychiatrists. Baldur von Schirach, who greeted the news in amazement, said, "Well, that's the end of scientific psychology." Goering, seeing that Hess was now the center of attraction and enjoying it immensely, soon lost his pleasure at the joke of Hess's amnesia-faking.[4]

It is not the suggestion here that the custodial officer or any other jail attendant who is especially adept at detecting malingering should supplant the psychiatrist or psychologist as the expert on an accused's fitness to stand trial. The point is that fitness to stand trial can be measured by an ordinary view. Psychiatric examination does not further the inquiry. For a literal application of the test, the judge can by himself make as valid a decision as anyone on the basis of a few ordinary and simple questions put to the defendant.

Does the Actual Operation of the Test Correspond to Its Literal Interpretation?

In actual operation, it is clear that the rule on triability is often used for purposes other than that for which it was intended. It is used by defense attorneys to avoid a capital or life-imprisonment penalty, to delay a trial until the emotions of the prosecuting witnesses and the public have calmed, or until memories have faded, so that the prosecuting attorney cannot prove the case "beyond a reasonable doubt."

In recent years, however, more and more defense lawyers have hesitated to raise the issue because it results in a distinct disadvantage to the accused. If the accused has a heart condition or other physical disability which results in a continuance or postponement of a trial, he is not restrained in his movement, assuming he has bail. However, one found incompetent to stand trial on account of mental disease or defect is automatically confined, whatever the offense, in a unit for the criminally insane, which is invariably located in a remote part of the state. As a result of the plea, the accused is placed for an indeterminable period of time in a facility which has the poorest conditions and carries the greatest stigma. A Massachusetts law enacted in 1971 requiring that criminal defendants be screened by psychiatrists on an out-patient basis before they can be committed if their competence to stand trial is questioned has reportedly led to a 50 percent cut in pretrial commitments to state mental institutions.

Today, the issue is raised as frequently by the prosecuting attorney or the court on its own motion as by defense counsel. The Supreme Court has ruled that when there is evidence that the defendant is incompetent to stand trial, the court must, on its own motion, hold a hearing to determine this issue, for to try an incompetent defendant is to deny him due process of law.[5] Thus, paradoxically, a doctrine which arose for the benefit of the accused has been turned against him; but not without good reason.

Quite frequently, the prosecuting attorney or the judge raises the issue of the accused's unfitness to proceed so as to accomplish the goal of preventive or long-term detention which otherwise would not be available under the criminal-law process. The criminal charge serves as little more than a fictional jurisdictional excuse for indeterminate confinement. In reaching this decision the court calls for a psychiatric evaluation of the defendant, since both the nature of the defendant's personality as well as the nature of the alleged offense are considerations. More often than not, however, the court uses the psychiatric report to justify what it wants to do about the defendant. If it disagrees with the evaluation, the court may appoint a different commission to examine the defendant, and it is not unheard of for several commissions to be appointed within a span of a few weeks. The prohibition against double jeopardy, which provides that a person shall not be twice put on trial for the same offense, does not apply to pretrial proceedings. Eventually, the court will obtain the desired report. The report is typically window dressing, but a judicial decision needs dressing.

Often a case arises where the accused is grossly psychotic but his alleged offense is of a minor nature. For example, commitment may not be available for a man who, without any apparent rational purpose, brutally stabs a cow to death; the hospital may not want him, or civil commitment procedures may not be within the jurisdiction of prosecuting officials. Achieving the goal of long-term or preventive detention through the triability issue may therefore be considered justified in order to protect society. Assuming *pro argumendo,* that the individual is dangerous, it still may be questioned whether the method by which detention is accomplished is either honest or helpful.

Although units for the criminally insane confine some dangerous persons, those detained are primarily mental defectives, usually harmless but bothersome persons. The community does not know how else to deal with them, nor do they know how to exist in the community. Consider, for example, the typical case of the person who makes a nuisance of himself by window peeping or lowering his pants in public. He is generally arrested on a charge of vagrancy or disorderly conduct which carries a light penalty. As he is usually of low intelligence, however, he will never be able to understand a trial or to assist counsel. As experience teaches that peepers and exhibitionists are usually repeaters, and because he is often without friends or funds, he spends the rest of his days forgotten in a colony for the criminally insane. His chance of ever being put to trial is rare. Should a trial occur, time spent in pretrial commitment need not be credited toward sentence.[6]

The mental defective is one whose capacity to stand trial will not improve. His subnormal mentality will be with him to the end of his days.[7] Others in a similar dilemma include those suffering from amnesia. Theoretically, capacity to stand trial includes the ability on the part of the accused to recall events so that his counsel can be furnished the facts necessary for the preparation of his defense. The test of competency to stand trial has been expressed by one court as whether the defendant "is possessed of sufficient mental power and has such understanding of his situation, such coherency of ideas, control of his mental faculties, and the requisite power of memory, as will enable him to testify in his own behalf . . . and otherwise to properly and intelligently aid his counsel in making a rational defense."[8]

Some individuals may react to the emotional trauma of committing a crime with a process of forgetting whereby memory is never revived. A passive individual who on a rare occasion bursts out in anger is apt to block out all recollection of the commission of a crime. Recollection via sodium amytal may be unwarranted because of the possibility of psychotic breakdown. Some individuals may have no recollection of behavior committed while under the influence of alcohol. A defendant who has alcoholic amnesia is generally found fit to stand trial since it is not "a result of a mental disease or defect."[9]

Deaf-mutes are commonly found fit for trial. Recently, in a particularly difficult case in Illinois, an accused who could not hear, speak, read, or write, was charged with the fatal stabbing and beating of a woman friend. Since, in addition, he did not understand sign language, not only was he unable to understand what was happening at the trial, but he was also unable to communicate with his attorney. He was found mentally and physically incompetent to stand trial and was sent to a state school. The authorities there reported that the accused "resists all efforts to teach him to communicate but is in all other respects of average intelligence." The Illinois Supreme Court pondered: Was it legally justified in confining the accused to a state institution indefinitely, when he had neither been convicted of a crime nor judged insane? It was shown that before the killing the accused had lived with his relatives and in no way represented a threat to others or to himself. Since the state was unwilling to free him outright, his attorney preferred the risks of trial to the near certainty of confinement for life. The Illinois Supreme Court, in ruling that the accused was competent to stand trial, ostensibly based its decision on the ground that the accused was physically incompetent and thereby eluded the statute which applied only to those who are mentally incompetent.[10]

In cases where the triability issue is raised, there is something about the nature of the offense or the nature of the defendant himself which prompts its invocation or application. Rudolf Hess and a number of run-of-the-mill cases have been mentioned. The most widely publicized are exceptional cases with political implications, as those involving Major General Edwin A. Walker, Dr. Robert Soblen, and poet Ezra Pound. Sentiment toward the defendant determined disposition.

Major General Edwin A. Walker had commanded the federal troops in the 1957 desegregation crisis at Little Rock. In 1961, he resigned from the U.S. Army, and in 1962, when federal troops were sent to the University of Mississippi to enforce James Meredith's enrollment, he went to Oxford allegedly to aid Mississippi segregationists. The Government charged him with several offenses but then sought to have him declared incompetent to stand trial. Federal District Judge Claude Clayton felt constrained to order a psychiatric examination, even though, on the basis of his own information and observation, he considered Walker fit to stand trial. Following hearings in November, 1968, the court declared him fit to stand trial. In his memorandum, giving the reasons for his decision, Judge Clayton spoke of Walker as follows:

. . . it would be improper for me to express my personal views—I do think, however, it would be proper for me to say that I know his career as a soldier and as an officer personally to a much greater extent than has been developed in the record here. I have long admired the character of his service in that capacity. I had, and still have, the greatest respect for him for that outstanding service in which he followed the flag wherever duty called.[11]

Somewhat earlier in the course of the hearings, Judge Clayton is quoted as having remarked:

[F]rom the appearance of Edwin A. Walker on the witness stand, his response to the questions put by counsel, from a layman's standpoint as distinguished from the psychiatric standpoint, if I had limited my consideration to that and that alone, on a hearing where I had to make a judicial determination thereof, I would necessarily have found, as I am sure most of you would have, that this man is competent within the meaning of the statute, capable of advising and assisting his counsel in the preparation of his defense in such criminal charges as may be presented against him by the Grand Jury of this Court.[12]

The Government thereupon dismissed its cases against Walker.

Dr. Robert Soblen, charged with treason as a Soviet spy, sought a continuance by raising the incompetency plea probably in order to ride out the anti-Communist hysteria of the times. Suffering from incurable lymphatic leukemia, he contended that necessary medication caused him to sleep through the trial proceedings and, thus, on appeal argued, without success, that he should not have been put to trial. He spent most of the trial curled up in a special contour chair rented by the court. Most of the time his eyes were closed. When the case reached trial, Dr. Soblen's condition had deteriorated, and he could not function in the courtroom without the administration of drugs and sedatives, including Demerol, Thorazine, and other tranquilizers. He also received cortisone preparations both before and during the trial. Dr. Soblen was frequently in great pain throughout the trial due to pressure of the enlarged spleen and enlarged liver which frequently made sitting difficult. Toward the end of the trial his condition worsened to such a degree that it was necessary for him to lie on a couch in the courtroom, which he did by leave of court. He was in a sleepy state during a great part of the trial and was frequently, even when awake, unable to follow the trial proceeding. While he was physically present, albeit in a horizontal position, his state of mind, induced by required sedation, made him mentally absent. His plea of incompetency to stand trial was not upheld, however, and he was convicted.[13]

Poet Ezra Pound, who spent World War II broadcasting for Mussolini, was found mentally unfit to face treason charges, and he spent thirteen years in the criminal ward of St. Elizabeth's Hospital in Washington, D.C. A board of psychiatrists appointed by the court gave their unanimous opinion that Pound was mentally unfit to advise counsel properly or to participate intelligibly in his own defense. Had he been tried, he would have insisted on testifying that America's entry into the war was a conspiracy between Roosevelt and the Jews and that, in opposing such a war over the Italian radio, he had acted to save the U.S. Constitution. His attorney, Thurman Arnold, says that it would have been an injustice to Pound to go to trial until he had been cured of his delusions and no longer insistent upon testifying in his own behalf. At the very beginning, however, it was apparent to the staff at St. Elizabeth's, judging from his inability to cooperate with his counsel, that Pound was incurably insane.[14]

Pound's long detention in the criminal ward of St. Elizabeth's Hospital aroused the ire of the literary world here and abroad. During his confinement he wrote his masterful *Pisan Cantos* and was awarded the 1949 Bollingen Prize. According to Arnold, no one in the Department of Justice wanted to keep him confined, but there seemed to be no way of getting him out once he was in. The fact that he was "too mentally ill to be tried" was not a reason for releasing him because this had nothing to do with his insanity at the time of the offense. He could not be pardoned because he had not been convicted of any offense. He could not be tried and acquitted on the ground of insanity, because he refused to make that defense, and he could not legally be forced to make it. Arnold was of the opinion that had Mrs. Pound, acting as Pound's guardian, asked for habeas corpus on the ground that it was absurd to confine Pound for life because he could not be tried, she might have succeeded, though this had been tried once and failed, in the lower court. Thus there was no way, in conformity with the legal logic of the situation, to release Pound other than dismissal of the indictment by the prosecution. Reflecting on the case, Arnold writes:

. . . The only way to liberate Pound without offending the logic of the law was to dismiss the indictment. This the Attorney General declined to do, for understandable reasons. To take affirmative action liberating a man who had broadcast against the United States in time of war, and who in addition was a notorious anti-Semite, would have put the Department of Justice under sharp attack. . . . [P]erhaps while the Attorney General would not affirmatively dismiss the indictment, he would not oppose a motion to dismiss it if I made it.[15]

Arnold took the chance and filed the motion, which succeeded. He supported the motion with an affidavit from Dr. Winfred Overholser, Superintendent of St. Elizabeth's, saying that Pound was insane and could never be in a position to stand trial, and that he would not be dangerous if released. In what has come to be known as an admirable pronouncement, Dr. Overholser said that "Pound is not too dangerous to go free in his wife's care, and too insane ever to be tried."[16]

In contrast to other states, Michigan has legislation placing an eighteen-month limitation on commitment to the criminally insane unit.[17] With the advent of pharmaceutical drugs, individuals whose capacity to stand trial will improve will do so in a relatively short period; otherwise, their condition is likely to be permanent, and they should be in a place other than the criminally insane unit. As far as security is concerned, prison offers more protection than these institutions. There are available for individuals not found ready for trial but who are not dangerous, special institutions for the mentally retarded or defective, as well as the state mental hospital.[18]

Indeed, there is no need for the criminally insane unit or maximum security hospital. They have fallen into obsolescence. In addition to perpetuating existing problems, these institutions prevent needed changes and reforms which can ultimately benefit all groups of inmates regardless of their particular status relative to the law. Dr. C. B. Scrignar, who has been a consultant at the security hospital in Louisiana for a period of years, suggests that the problems of defendants, patients, or prisoners can be simplified by the following formula: If treatment is of primary concern and security secondary, this category of patients can be treated in the public mental hospital; if security is of primary importance, psychiatric treatment can occur in the appropriate jail, prison, or penitentiary. The defendants adjudicated not guilty because of insanity, who are few in number, can in most cases be treated in a civil hospital where security, seclusion, or confinement can be applied whenever necessary. This is the same formula as for those patients who have no legal status.[19]

On the basis of the author's extensive interviews with inmates at criminal insane units, it appears that almost half the persons committed as untriable meet the test of triability as ordinarily understood. Of the other half, approximately half (or 25 percent of the total) consists of persons who could meet the test if they were maintained on pharmacological drugs. The remaining 25 percent are persons who, by reason of mental defect or amnesia, will never literally be in a position to assist counsel. The conclusion is obvious that the rule on triability is generally misapplied in order to confine the accused for an indeterminate period because he is dangerous or a nuisance. There are situations in which the hospital defers recommending the inmate back to court because he is dangerous; usually, however, the court fails to respond to overtures from the hospital that the individual is able to stand trial. There is no law authorizing the hospital on its own initiative to return the accused to the local jailhouse from whence he came or to discharge persons accused of crime. Local jailhouses are crowded, and the cost of confinement is shifted from the municipality to the state by confinement in the state hospital. The hospital is usually located outside the jurisdiction of a legal-aid society, and the persons committed generally do not have funds to hire an attorney.

There is confusion in many states as to whether the prosecuting attorney or the judge has the responsibility for the individual once he has been sent to the hospital. In the case of long commitments, it invariably occurs that a new judge occupies the bench or that the case is forgotten by the court. Witnesses move away; new prosecutors come along; sometimes even the records are lost. A decade or even more may pass with no action taken on a letter. To illustrate, from hospital files, the hospital writes to the court: "The patient has been at the hospital now for about 24 years and since we have informed him that he meets the test of triability, you can understand his eager anticipation and his disappointment resulting from this delay." The judge in due course replies: "This will acknowledge receipt of your letter. Because of my involvement in long and tedious cases I was unable to reply sooner. I will acquaint myself with the record in this case, and as soon as I have enough information to express an opinion, I will let you hear from me." In this case, several years later, the patient remains at the security unit of the hospital and will probably die there.

There are even times when no one knows why an individual is committed to the security area of the hospital. Again from hospital files, the hospital writes to the judge and the district attorney for clarification: "We would appreciate having a statement clarifying the patient's legal status and informing us as to what disposition might be made of the patient." There is no word from the court; the district attorney in this case replied: "After a check of the records of this district, I am unable to find any charges pending against him in this district. I suggest you check with district attorneys in other parts of the State." The case thus far has been going round and round for seven years.

There may be collaboration or collusion between judge and prosecuting attorney in which the judge initially stalls and then finds out from the prosecuting attorney that his office does not want the man back in the community. Again from hospital files, the hospital writes to the judge: "It is our belief that the patient can understand proceedings and cooperate with counsel in the preparation and conduct of his defense. It is therefore respectfully requested of the Honorable Court that deputies with your written permission be dispatched, so that we may turn our patient over to their custody so that the patient may be returned to the Honorable Court." Some weeks later the judge advised the hospital: "It was our purpose to answer your letter much more promptly; however, in this case we did not want to give a directive until we conferred with the district attorney's office. It is not always possible to catch the proper officer in the office, and we were somewhat delayed in getting the final conference. After referring the above matter to the district attorney, we were advised that their office does not want this man back in the community."

Although the court may make a point of seeking out a psychiatrist or appointing a lunacy commission, ostensibly for the professional opinion they can bring to bear on the case, the psychiatrist may find himself used as a cover behind which the court and prosecuting attorney do as they please. The opinion of the psychiatrist is irrelevant in cases where the judge or prosecuting attorney believes that the accused is a nuisance or is dangerous and ought to be locked up, or where there is the possibility of capital punishment, and the judge or prosecuting attorney is opposed to it. There are cases of commitment on grounds of incapacity to stand trial, notwithstanding the opinion of the lunacy commission and that of the defense counsel. In many of these cases, the defendant is better versed in the criminal law and able to defend himself better than the neophyte criminal lawyer. Even paranoid individuals, who probably make the best defense, should have their day in court.

The triability issue is an illustration of the use of language to achieve a purpose other than the one expressed. It is an illustration of people saying one thing and meaning another. When a psychiatrist is called for an expert opinion, the court really does not want to know whether or not the accused is capable of standing trial; it wants to know whether the accused is likely to be dangerous or unduly bothersome in the community. In other words, labeling a person "incompetent to stand trial" signifies that he is either dangerous or a nuisance. Thus, to focus on the literal meaning of the triability test is to engage in a metaphysical exercise.

This comes out clearly in the difficulties encountered by the superintendent of the criminally insane unit who certifies to the court that a defendant is "competent to stand trial" under a literal interpretation of the test but who is still maintained on tranquilizers. Refusal to accept for trial a defendant who is competent only with the aid of pharmacological drugs clearly indicates that the judge is concerned not with the defendant's capacity to undergo trial but with his ability to get along without drugs. Parenthetically: Albert Speer surreptitiously took a tranquilizer upon being called to the stand at the Nuremberg trials; he says in his memoirs, *Inside the Third Reich:* "When I went to the witness stand, I had stage fright. I hastily swallowed a tranquilizing pill the German doctor had prudently handed to me."

At the same time that the general public is extensively using drugs as medication, and hyperactive school children are being calmed with amphetamines, the judge in these competency cases is concerned that the accused, an individual who has already shown himself—albeit allegedly —to be troublesome to the community, may not continue pharmacological treatment in the event of release.

The real significance of triability is also apparent when it is considered that the issue does not hold up civil cases. Furthermore, in a criminal trial, the defendant is not required to put on any proof of his innocence; the state has the burden of proving beyond a reasonable doubt the defendant's guilt. Moreover, the usual criminal case does not go to trial. Rather, perhaps as many as 95 percent of the cases are resolved, not by a full presentation of the evidence at trial, but by a private plea-bargaining process between the prosecutor and defense lawyer. Admittedly, it should be important to the defense attorney to be able to obtain all the facts from his client before he decides whether plea-bargaining is the best alternative. The plea-bargaining process in practice, however, is not frustrated because the accused is unable to relate all meaningful facts. The prime considerations in the plea-bargaining process are the character and criminal record of the accused, not his guilt, of which there is usually strong evidence. In the usual case, the defense lawyer spends little time with the defendant; his ambition each day is to enter several pleas of guilty, at $50–$100 each. Hence, to speak about competency for trial is to talk about a metaphysical trial. The fact that the triability issue is mainly raised by the prosecutor further undermines the theoretical justification of the plea of incompetency-to-stand-trial.[20]

What Is the Relevance of the Courtroom Decorum Cases?

In recent years a new aspect of the incompetency issue has arisen in the so-called courtroom decorum cases. In these cases, tactics of disruption have turned trials into spectacles of disorder and even violence. These tactics, involving contemptuous language and other techniques, appear deliberately designed by the defendant (and tolerated and encouraged by some counsel) to frustrate the judicial process. During the Chicago conspiracy trial in 1969, the trial judge ordered physical restraints (gags and shackles) on former Harlem theater actor Bobby Seale, a procedure upheld by the Court of Appeals because "no other remedy was available to the trial judge."[21]

A year later, the Supreme Court in *Illinois v. Allen* (a rare unanimous decision) stated that a judge must maintain decorum in his courtroom and may use *any* means to restrain an obstreperous defendant or witness, including handcuffs, gags, or removal from the room.[22] Such a procedure is necessary, Justice Black said, to show that "our courts . . . cannot be treated disrespectfully with impunity." In this case, the accused, whose mental competence was questionable, had initially refused appointed counsel in his robbery trial. During the voir-dire examination of the jury, he argued with the judge in a most abusive and disrespectful manner. He said, "When I go out for lunchtime you [the judge] are going to be a corpse here." At that point he tore up his attorney's file, scattered the pieces on the courtroom floor, and twice announced his intention to prevent any proceedings against him.

In the course of upholding the trial court for excluding the defendant from the courtroom when his behavior was contumacious, Justice Black wrote: "Although mindful that courts must indulge every reasonable presumption against the loss of constitutional rights . . . we explicitly hold today that a defendant can lose his right to be present at trial if, after he has been warned by the judge that he will be removed if he continues his disruptive behavior, he nevertheless insists on conducting himself in a manner so disorderly, disruptive, and disrespectful of the court that his trial cannot be carried on with him in the courtroom."[23]

Is an exception to the prohibition against trials in absentia to be made only when the defendant has apparent control over his behavior? In such a case it may be said that, if the defendant wants to be present, he has an easy choice: he can decide to behave. But such an option is not available to the person who is mentally "out of it." The Court in *Allen* ruled as it did notwithstanding the questionable mental competence of the defendant. In condoning trial in absentia, the Court implied that there are no longer any substantial societal interests underlying the defendant's ancient right to be present and that exceptions to the general prohibition against trials in absentia might be developed or expanded.

In early common law the accused did not have the right to testify because it was considered that his interest in the outcome of the case would cause him to twist his tongue. He had a right to confront the witnesses and to cross-question them without the aid of counsel. In early English procedure, a person charged with treason or a felony (of which there were over 160) was denied the assistance of counsel. Lord Coke defended the rule on the ground that in felonies the court itself was counsel for the accused. In 1836, Parliament permitted representation by counsel in felony cases. The American Bill of Rights provides that "In all criminal prosecutions, the accused shall enjoy the right . . . to be confronted with the witnesses against him," and rejecting the early English common-law rule, it also provides the right "to have the Assistance of Counsel for his defence."

Subtracting the assistance of counsel, the defendant's presence is essential if he is to utilize the right to cross-question witnesses. But, in the United States, the defendant is entitled to counsel, and in the case of indigency, is assigned counsel. Given the assistance of counsel, the defendant's presence is diminished in importance. Justice Cardozo once observed: "Confusion of thought will result if we fail to make the distinction between requirements in respect of presence that have their source in common law, and the requirements that have their source, either expressly or by implication, in the federal constitution. Confusion will result again if the privilege of presence be identified with the privilege of confrontation."[24]

Generally speaking, an accused has the right to dispense with counsel and to represent himself, but this right is subject to the duty of the court to protect the judicial process from deterioration occasioned by improper or inadequate conduct of the defense. The court can impose counsel on an accused against his will, not only when he is obstreperous but also when it appears that he is mentally incompetent or for some reason incapable of conducting his own defense. The role of the psychiatrist in detecting malingering or administering tranquilizing medication raises unresolved legal questions.

CONCLUSION

It may be concluded that the triability issue—and the unit for the criminally insane which implements it—has little merit and can be eliminated. Anything accomplished in such units apparently can be better accomplished through the ordinary criminal-law process and civil-commitment procedures. It is argued, however, that some flexible method is needed to deal with troublesome individuals who, for one reason or another, escape these processes. Until something better comes along, the triability issue has this pragmatic appeal, but it can adversely affect the process of administering justice in terms of confidence in the system. As in measuring a "just war," the test apparently is whether the good results exceed the bad.

NOTES

1. *Dusky v. United States*, 362 U.S. 402 (1960). See also *People v. Burson*, 11 Ill.2d 360, 143 N.E.2d 239 (1957). As the time-of-trial incompetency issue is one of procedure rather than substance, i.e., does not bear on the question of guilt or innocence, a jury trial on the issue is not a requirement. Nor does the privilege against self-incrimination bar a psychiatric evaluation of the accused on the issue. See Comment, *Harv. L. Rev.* 83:648, 1970.
2. One psychiatrist, indeed, one frequently appointed to serve as an examiner and thus experienced, at a hearing to determine the accused's mental capacity to proceed testified:
   Q. Doctor, are you familiar with the test a defendant in a criminal proceeding like this must pass before he can be adjudged to be able to stand trial?
   A. You mean the M'Naughten Rule test? I am familiar with it, yes.
   Q. If I may read to you . . . the Code of Criminal Procedure . . . (which) says "Mental incapacity to proceed exists when as a result of mental disease or defect, a defendant presently lacks the capacity to," now, this is the important phrase, in my opinion, "to understand the proceedings against or to assist in his defense." Now is that the M'Naughten Rule?
   A. That is my understanding. Yes.
   Q. Doctor, in your opinion, would you apply the rule to the defendant? That rule.
   A. I think that he is able to understand right and wrong. I am not sure that he is able to understand the complete nature of the offense.
   [Brief of Defendant-Appellant, *Louisiana v. Edwards*, 257 La. 707, 243 So.2d 806 (1971).]
      There are some twenty-eight different legal tests of capacity, each of which relates to a specific legal operation. Mezer, R. R., and Rheingold, P. D.   The Use of Psychiatry in Mental Competency Cases. *Boston Bar J.*, Dec. 1961, p. 10; Role of the Psychiatrist in Mental Competency Cases. *Prac. Law.* 9:85, 1963. To take another example, an unborn child is considered a "person" in some situations but not in others. [*O'Neill v. Morse*, 20 Mich. App. 699, 174 N.W.2d 575 (1969).]
3. *Pouncey v. United States*, 349 F.2d 699, 701 (D.C. Cir. 1965).
4. Gilbert, G. M. *Nuremberg Diary*. New York: Signet Books, 1947. Pp. 52–53. Gilbert (now Chairman of the Department of Psychology at Long Island University) says that during the course of the trial Hess became amnesic again. He suffered, Gilbert says, from recurrent or hysterical amnesia. Gilbert says that he could shake up Hess by calling him non compos mentis; Hess did not like being called crazy. Gilbert reported Hess as competent to stand trial because he was able, during his lucid intervals, to confer with his counsel. Although Gilbert felt that it was important to be especially careful in the evaluation of the accused at Nuremberg because it was an international trial, he reported Hess competent to stand trial notwithstanding his recurrent amnesia. [Conversation with author on February 24, 1971.]
      Douglas McGladen Kelley, a psychiatrist nationally known as an authority on

Rorschach testing, who along with Gilbert was assigned to observe the Nuremberg prisoners, contended that Rudolf Hess's amnesia was not a hoax and that his claim that it was a pretense was untrue. See Kelley, D. M. *22 Cells at Nuremberg: A Psychiatrist Examines the Nazi Criminals.* New York: Greenberg, 1947. See also his Preliminary Studies of the Rorschach Records of the Nazi War Criminals. *Rorschach Research Exchange* 10:45, 1946. Kelley was present at Nuremberg in the pretrial stage and only during the first month of the trial. He returned to the United States and shortly thereafter committed suicide in the same manner as Goering.

5. *Pate v. Robinson,* 383 U.S. 375 (1966); *Bishop v. United States,* 350 U.S. 961 (1956). In *Pate,* the defendant, charged with the murder of his common-law wife, introduced evidence that he was incompetent but failed to request a hearing on that issue as required under state law, relying instead on his insanity-at-time-of-offense plea. On appeal, the prosecutor urged that the competency issue had been waived below. The Supreme Court ruled that the trial court's failure to conduct a hearing on the competency issue on its own initiative was a denial of due process and this issue is not waived by counsel's failure to raise it at trial. In the *Bishop* case, the defendant was convicted in 1938 of murder in the first degree and sentenced to death. Prior to trial a psychiatrist had examined the defendant at the insistence of the U.S. Attorney and found him to be of low intelligence but not of sufficient degree to affect his responsibility. The defendant in 1940 was adjudged insane and sent to a hospital. In May 1952 the President commuted the sentence to life imprisonment; in November 1952 the accused was certified to have recovered his reason and was returned to prison. He then made a motion to vacate the judgment of conviction on the ground, among others, that he was not mentally competent to stand trial in 1938. The district court considered the evidentiary material in the record, made a finding of the defendant's competency to have stood trial, and denied the motion to vacate. The Supreme Court ordered the district court to hold a hearing on the sanity of the defendant at the time of his trial. See Notes, *Vill. L. Rev.* 12:655, 1967; *W. Va. L. Rev.* 58:94, 1955.

6. The Illinois and Michigan statutes are atypical in providing prison credit for the time spent at the mental institution. [*Ill. Rev. Stat.* ch. 38, §104-3 (1967); *Mich. Comp. Laws Ann.* §767.27a(9) (1968).]

7. A person, for example, 18 years of age with an I.Q. level of 59 and a mental age of 8 or 9 years would have the understanding of about an 8- or 9-year-old child and could reason with about the same ability. He would understand what was going on only to a limited degree and might not say the things that would be in his best interest. His capacity to assist counsel is never going to change. While the argument is logical that such a mentally retarded person should not be tried for a crime any more than an actual child of nine years, it has never been accepted by the courts. See Person, J. P. The Accused Retardate. *Colum. Survey of Human Rights Law* 4:239, 1972.

8. *United States v. Chisolm,* 149 Fed. 284 (S.D. Ala. 1906). See Koson, D., and Robey, A. Amnesia and Competency to Stand Trial. *Am. J. Psychiatry* 130:588, 1973.

9. *State v. Palmer,* 232 La. 468, 94 So.2d 439 (1957).

10. *People ex rel. Myers v. Briggs,* 46 Ill.2d 281, 263 N.E.2d 109 (1970), noted in *U. Ill. L. For.* 1971:278; *Time,* Jan. 11, 1971, p. 51. An interesting aspect of the competency problem arises in connection with transfers of jurisdiction from juvenile to criminal courts and trying the juvenile as an adult. The juvenile laws of a number of jurisdictions recognize that certain extreme conduct necessitates different handling and provide "vents" for the system, by allowing transfer of juveniles to the regular criminal courts. In order to "transfer" or "waive" juvenile-court jurisdiction, certain criteria such as age, nature of the crime, and prior record have to be met. In *Kent v. United States,* 401 F.2d 408 (D.C. Cir. 1968), the juvenile appealed the juvenile court's waiver of jurisdiction to criminal court,

arguing that he was incompetent to be sent over to the criminal court because he was schizophrenic. Judge Bazelon, writing the opinion, stated that it is implicit in the juvenile-court scheme that no criminal treatment is to be the rule—and the adult criminal treatment, the exception which must be governed by the particular factors of individual cases. On the facts of this case waiver was inappropriate. The theory of allowing insanity as a defense to waiver is in accord with the prevailing philosophy of the juvenile court. Judge Bazelon wrote: "Since waiver was not necessary for the protection of society and not conducive to [appellant's] rehabilitation, its exercise in this case violated the social welfare philosophy of the Juvenile Court Act. Of course, this philosophy does not forbid all waivers. We only decide here that it does forbid waivers of a seriously ill juvenile." [401 F.2d at 412.] Judge Burger, now Chief Justice of the Supreme Court, vigorously dissented. The main reason for waivers is that the juvenile court retains jurisdiction over a juvenile offender for a few years, until he reaches majority, and he may remain a danger when twenty-one. Comments, *Baylor L. Rev.* 21:333, 1969; *Colum. L. Rev.* 68:1149, 1968; *Ohio St. L.J.* 31:623, 1970; *Wis. L. Rev.* 1966:866. "Insanity" as a defense in a juvenile court proceeding was reviewed in a New Jersey case, which held that a juvenile could be adjudicated a delinquent even though insane. The court noted the distinction between a juvenile case and an indictable offense; the focus in a juvenile proceeding is not upon the commission of the act itself but upon the consequences of it. In drawing this distinction, the court noted that an adjudication of delinquency brought about the protective and rehabilitative interests of the court. *In re State in Interest of H.C.*, 106 N.J. Super. 583, 256 A.2d 322 (1969). But see *In re M.G.S., a Minor*, 72 Cal. Rptr. 808 (1969).

11. Szasz, T. S. *Psychiatric Justice.* P. 219.
12. *Id.* at 220.
13. *National Observer*, Sept. 17, 1962; Brief of Amici Curiae in support of petition for writ of certiorari in *Soblen v. United States*, 301 F.2d 236 (2d Cir. 1962), *cert. denied*, 370 U.S. 944 (1962). While on bail pending an application for a new trial, Dr. Soblen flew, in June, 1962, to Israel. He was sent back to the United States; on the way he badly wounded himself with a knife in the aircraft. Following treatment in a London hospital, the Home Secretary ordered his deportation. Appealing unsuccessfully, he committed suicide.
14. Arnold, T. *Fair Fights and Foul.* P. 236.
15. *Id.* at 237.
16. *Id.* at 241. The question of whether to honor Pound as a poet is discussed in Howe, I. The Return of the Case of Ezra Pound. *World*, Oct. 24, 1972, p. 20.
17. The law provides, in part: "If after the defendant has been committed to its custody . . . the department of mental health believes that the defendant cannot recover competence to stand trial within eighteen months from the entry of the order of commitment, or if, by the expiration of eighteen months from the entry of the order of commitment, the defendant has not regained competence to stand trial in the opinion of the department of mental health, the department shall certify its opinion, together with a detailed psychiatric report, to the probate court from which the defendant was originally committed." [*Mich. Comp. Laws Annot.* §767.27a(7) (1968).]
18. Under the Michigan law, if the department of mental health is of the opinion that the accused will not be competent to stand trial within eighteen months from the time of commitment, it certifies this finding to the probate court in the county in which the defendant was committed, and the probate court proceeds with committing the individual as though it were a civil commitment under the civil commitment laws. If the probate court should decide to commit, there is no provision that the charges against the accused must be dropped with prejudice against the state. The statute of limitations does not run against the state when it is unable to prosecute. Therefore, if and when the individual should ever be discharged from the hospital, he theoretically could be arrested again for the crime. If the probate court

should decide not to commit, then it must transfer the case to the original committing court. Should that court find that the individual is still incompetent to stand trial, the order of the probate court is reversed and the individual is committed to the department of mental health for treatment in an appropriate state hospital. Here again there is no provision that the charges would be dismissed with prejudice.

19. Scrignar, C.   Maximum Security Hospitals: Where the People Are. *Newsletter,* American Academy of Psychiatry and Law, vol. 11, no. 3, April 1971. See also Slovenko, R.   The Criminally Insane Unit. *Am. Crim. L.Q.* 7:96, 1969. In the first half of the nineteenth century, accused offenders unable to stand trial, or those found not guilty by reason of insanity, or mentally ill prisoners, were committed to public hospitals. This was done, for example, at Worcester State Hospital and Utica State Hospital. Because of objections to the association of the criminal and the non-criminal, some mental hospitals built special annexes for them. The creation of special institutions, geographically distant, was a development somewhat later. Broadmoor in England, which opened in 1863, is the best known of such institutions, although the Auburn Lunatic Asylum, adjoining the state prison in New York, established in 1859, predated it. Daniel M'Naughten, from whose trial emerged the famous M'Naughten rules, was committed to Bethlehem Hospital in 1843 and was transferred in 1864 to the newly opened Broadmoor, where he died a year later of heart and kidney disease.

A special unit for the criminally insane, like the special unit for the sexual psychopath, has little to warrant it. In Germany a special institution has been maintained to detain one man, Rudolf Hess, for war crimes. It is an expensive operation, but justified on moral or political grounds. Special institutions for the alcoholic, the aged, and juveniles are justified on remedial or therapeutic grounds. On the other hand, special institutions have not been built and are not justified for armed robbers, burglars, or bad-check writers. At what point is a special institution justified?

Not long ago attorney Frederick Wiseman produced a 16-mm documentary film, *Titicut Follies*, made in the Massachusetts Bridgewater State Mental Hospital for the Criminally Insane. Like others, this institution looks like a snake pit, what with its exposed pipes, naked lights, seatless toilets, peeling walls, and an atmosphere of dampness. The resemblance to a snake pit is heightened by the life of the place—people masturbating in open view on the grounds, standing on their heads, or campaigning for Fulton Sheen for President. Most of the time, the inmates simply sit cramped together in a small, airless room. Work and recreation are almost totally nonexistent. The question is: Is there a more appropriate place that can meet the need of institutionalizing the type of people who are in institutions like Bridgewater—at the same time being more humane toward them and protecting society? Even the briefest visit to one of these institutions would reveal their utter folly.

Many of the inmates are of low intelligence, and consequently there is actually nothing to treat in the medical sense. They need supervision, or a simple environment. The criminal charge for most of these individuals can be dropped, as is required in one or two states and as recommended by the distinguished attorney Thurman Arnold, in his book *Fair Fights and Foul.* They may be sent under civil commitment to the institution for persons who are retarded or defective, or in the case of a psychotic individual, to a mental hospital.

The Michigan Department of Mental Health recommended the phasing out of Ionia State Hospital, the criminally insane unit, as follows: "Ionia State Hospital should be phased out insofar as its present function is concerned. The responsibility for treating mentally ill offenders should be decentralized to the Regional State Mental Hospitals in accordance with the concept of the Community Mental Health Centers. Patients who cannot be discharged from the Ionia State Hospital should be transferred to these hospitals for treatment. They should be treated the same as other patients to the extent possible. The necessary changes in the state statutes should be made to permit this change." Michigan Department of Mental Health. *Special Report on the Program and Assignment of the Ionia State Hospital, Including Recommendation for Immediate and Long-Range Changes.* Jan. 1966, p. 2.

Following the Supreme Court's decision in *Baxstrom v. Herold*, 383 U.S. 107 (1966), the New York Department of Mental Hygiene transferred to civil state hospitals all ex-prisoners whose sentences had expired and who were being held at Dannemora and Matteawan correctional hospitals. Baxstrom was a mentally ill convict who had been transferred from prison to Dannemora during his sentence, and upon expiration of that sentence he brought a writ of habeas corpus. In accordance with the Court's decision, he was admitted to the civil hospital as an involuntary patient following observance of civil commitment procedures on notice and hearing. This "Operation Baxstrom," as the transfer process has come to be denominated, argues against the existence of special correctional hospitals. The transfer of Baxstrom-type inmates, and discharge, as shown in follow-up studies has proved remarkably uneventful. Had it been suggested prior to the decision that this number of inmates should be transferred to civil mental hospitals or discharged it would have been considered impractical and unrealistic, but the transfers and subsequent discharges were made without any disastrous consequences. Morris, G. H. "Criminality" and the Right to Treatment. *U. Chi. L. Rev.* 36:784, 1969; Steadman, H. J., and Keveles, G. The Community Adjustment and Criminal Activity of the Baxstrom Patients. *Am. J. Psychiatry* 129: 304, 1972.

20. In cases where a trial is continued or postponed because of the accused's physical inability to stand trial (e.g., pneumonia or heart condition), he is usually released on bail, but in the case of incompetency due to mental disability, he is committed to an institution for the criminally insane. Most states by statute (e.g., Alabama, Arizona, California, Connecticut, Georgia, Indiana, Minnesota, Missouri, Montana, Nevada, New Jersey, North Carolina, North Dakota, Ohio, Utah, Wisconsin) or by judicial practice impose automatic, indeterminate commitment following a finding of incompetency to stand trial. "The widespread practice of automatically committing defendants incompetent to stand trial reflects an unawareness that the policies controlling whether a trial should be delayed are distinct from those controlling whether a person should be involuntarily committed. As a result, many of the present commitments of incompetent defendants serve no legitimate interest of the state." [Note. *Harv. L. Rev.* 81:454, 461, 1967.]

The federal statute, 18 U.S.C. §4247, provides for confinement of an incompetent defendant to a federal security hospital only if the court finds that "if released, accused probably will endanger the safety of officers, the property, or other interests of the United States." [*United States v. Curry*, 410 F.2d 1372 (4th Cir. 1969).] A number of states similarly require a finding of dangerousness to justify pretrial commitment of an incompetent defendant (e.g., Iowa, Oklahoma, South Dakota, Idaho). A few states (e.g., Kansas, Oregon, Wisconsin) authorize release on parole from the institution notwithstanding the pending criminal charges. Typically, the confinement is not "relevant to the purpose of assuring the presence of that defendant" at a future trial but rather is justified to protect society against his proclivities. Compare *Stack v. Boyle*, 342 U.S. 1, 5 (1951) on the right to bail; 11 A.L.R. 3d 1385 (1967).

The U.S. Supreme Court recently ruled that the automatic commitment for an indefinite term of a criminal defendant found to be incompetent and unlikely to be restored to competence within a reasonably short period of time, without traditional civil commitment safeguards, deprives him of the equal protection of the laws, the right to bail, and the right to a speedy trial. In this case, a 27-year-old retarded deaf-mute with a mental age of 3 or 4 was charged with two robberies (purse snatching involving a total of $9). The trial court found him to be incompetent to assist in his own defense and summarily committed him to the state mental institution for an open-ended period. Based on the record, he would apparently have been confined for the rest of his life, since there is virtually no chance that he can ever be made competent. At the time of the Supreme Court's ruling, the detention had gone on for four years. The trial court found only that he was incompetent to stand trial; it did not find that he required either treatment or custodial care in a mental hospital to guard against harm to himself or others. For all other persons civilly committed under Indiana state law, such findings are required. [*Jackson v. State,* 253 Ind. 487, 255 N.E.2d 515, 516 (1970), noted in *Ind. Leg. For.* 4:566, 1971.] The Supreme Court said: "[D]ue process requires that the nature and duration of commitment bear some reasonable relation to the purpose for which the individual is committed. We hold, consequently, that a person charged by a State with a criminal offense who is committed solely on account of his incapacity to proceed to trial cannot be held more than the reasonable period of time necessary to determine whether there is a substantial probability that he will attain that capacity in the foreseeable future. If it is determined that this is not the case, then the State must either institute the customary civil commitment proceeding [under either the general civil commitment statutes or those for the commitment of the feebleminded] that would be required to commit indefinitely any other citizen, or release the defendant." [*Jackson v. Indiana,* 406 U.S. 715 (1972).]

The Supreme Court in *Jackson v. Indiana* expressed surprise that the state's commitment power has been so seldom the subject of litigation and seemed to invite litigation on its scope. It stated: "The States have traditionally exercised broad power to commit persons found to be mentally ill. The substantive limitations on the exercise of this power and the procedures for invoking it vary drastically among the States. The particular fashion in which the power is exercised —for instance, through various forms of civil commitment, defective delinquency laws, sexual psychopath laws, commitment of persons acquitted by reason of insanity—reflects different combinations of distinct bases for commitment sought to be vindicated. The bases that have been articulated include dangerousness to self, dangerousness to others, and the need for care or treatment or training. Considering the number of persons affected, it is perhaps remarkable that the substantive constitutional limitations on this power have not been more frequently litigated." [406 U.S. at 736 (1972).]

Given the growing dissatisfaction with the commitment process involving criminal offenders, the Court in a number of cases has set down constraints requiring the application of civil commitment safeguards. In *Humphrey v. Cady,* 405 U.S. 504 (1972), the Court ruled that commitment for compulsory treatment under the Wisconsin Sex Crimes Act, at least after the expiration of the initial commitment in lieu of sentence, is essentially equivalent to civil commitment, and consequently the individual has a right to determination whether he meets the standards for commitment. See also *McNeil v. Director, Patuxent Institution,* 407 U.S. 245 (1972); discussed in Prettyman, E. B. The Indeterminate Sentence and the Right to Treatment. *Am. Crim. L. Rev.* 11:7, 1972; *Specht v. Patterson,* 386 U.S. 605 (1967); *Baxstrom v. Herold,* 383 U.S. 107 (1966). See *Wilson v. State,* 287 N.E.2d 875 (Ind. 1972)—persons acquitted by reason of insanity are constitutionally entitled to the procedural guarantees afforded to those committed civilly.

Some states (e.g., New York) provide for jury trial of dangerousness for civil commitment. The Supreme Court recently ruled under the doctrine of equal protection that in criminal cases in those jurisdictions, a person too mentally ill to stand trial may not be confined for an extended period on account of dangerousness unless a jury likewise determines the issue. [*Gomez v. Miller,* 41 U.S.L.W. 3621 (May 29, 1973), affirming 341 F. Supp. 323 (S.D. N.Y. 1972).] The decision represents a departure from the traditional view that competency-to-stand-trial is a purely procedural question, reserved for the judge alone; and it represents another step toward ending the criminally insane unit.

See generally the report, a project supported by the National Institute of Mental Health from the Laboratory of Community Psychiatry of Harvard Medical School, by McGarry, A. L., et al. *Competency to Stand Trial and Mental Illness.* Washington, D.C.: U.S. Govt. Printing Office, 1973.

21. *Seale v. Hoffman,* 306 F. Supp. 330 (N.D. Ill. 1969).
22. 397 U.S. 337 (1970).
23. *Id.* at 343.
24. *Snyder v. Massachusetts,* 291 U.S. 97, 107 (1934); discussed in Note, *Cal. Western L. Rev.* 7:286, 1970. The right to cross-examination is an opportunity which may be waived. As Dean Wigmore, the leading commentator on the law of evidence, has put it: "The principle requiring a testing of testimonial statements by cross-examination has always been understood as requiring, not necessarily an actual cross-examination, but merely an opportunity to exercise the right to cross-examine if desired." Wigmore, J. *Evidence* §1371 (3d ed.). Boston: Little, Brown, 1940.

7. COMPETENCY TO BE EXECUTED

ACCORDING to the *Uniform Crime Reports* of the FBI, over 8,000 murders and 16,000 forcible rapes, long punishable by death, are committed each year in the United States. A number of these offenders are acquitted on the ground of insanity and thereupon committed to mental institutions to remain until no longer considered dangerous to society. Others are found guilty with recommendation of mercy and spend ten to fifteen years (the average time served under life sentence) in prison. Others have been sentenced to death.

During the 1960s juries returned some 2,000 death sentences. This is a significant number, to be sure, but it represents a minority of the capital cases before the courts during that period. In 1972 the Supreme Court rendered its highly publicized death penalty opinions, ruling 5-4 that the death penalty in its present form is unconstitutional. While no unifying reason supported the decision, the net result, with each Justice writing his own opinion (243 pages in all), was that the death penalty, as imposed within the discretion of juries, violates the Eighth Amendment, not because it is inherently intolerable, but because it is applied so rarely, "so wantonly and freakishly," that it serves no valid purpose and now constitutes cruel and unusual punishment. Only two justices—Justices Brennan and Marshall—ruled the death penalty unconstitutional per se. The dissenting justices felt that the majority had gone beyond judicial jurisdiction and trespassed upon the prerogatives of the legislature.[1]

Thus capital punishment in its present form was rendered "cruel and unusual" by operation of what was intended to be, at the time of its introduction, an ameliorative feature of the criminal justice system—the jury's discretion to impose a lesser sentence than death. The Court, finding no reason to believe that the death sentence was imposed with "informed selectivity," concluded that it was imposed in a way that arbitrarily and capriciously discriminated against minorities and the poor.

Chief Justice Warren Burger then touched on changes that would have to be made to allow the use of the death penalty in compliance with the result of the case. The Court implied that capital punishment would be sanctioned if the penalty is uniformly and consistently applied. Legislative enactment of mandatory death sentences would provide one answer. Justice Burger wrote: "Since there is no majority of the court on the ultimate issue presented in these cases, the future of capital punishment in this country has been left in an uncertain limbo."

The Supreme Court was concerned with the sentencing process, and not being called upon to do so, did not devote any attention to the posttrial phase of capital cases. The death penalty as far as actual implementation is concerned had already fallen into disuse at the time of the Court's decision. There had not been an execution in the United States since June 2, 1967, when Luis José Monge was put to death in the gas chamber at the Colorado State Prison for murdering his pregnant wife and three of their seven children. In 1965, there were seven executions; in 1966, one; in 1967, two; and since then, none. While the number of persons actually executed had been dropping steadily through the years, the number awaiting execution in 1972 had never been greater. At the time of the Court's decision, some 600 condemned prisoners (257 white and 343 black or other) had accumulated on the nation's death rows.

How did this extraordinary situation arise? Was it the result of illogical theory and slipshod methods? One criminologist has observed, "The public does not ordinarily realize how many different ways execution of the death sentence can be avoided." After the trial stage is completed in a capital case, as in other cases, the court machinery continues to operate for some time. The jury's decision is blocked by further litigation and seemingly endless hearings. Appeals are made at all levels of the state courts as well as the federal courts. In capital cases, though, American courts must be emphatically sure: "No man shall be executed while there is the slightest doubt either as to his guilt or as to the legality of the process by which his guilt was determined." Appeals courts carefully scanned the transcript; error was uncovered and deemed prejudicial which would have been overlooked in noncapital cases. New trials were regularly granted.

The courts were not commended, however, but bitterly criticized for their scrutiny of capital cases. It was said, "The whole procedure is insane"; "the lengthy procedure in capital cases is the enduring shame of American judicial procedure." These criticisms were commonplace because the basis of appeal or writ of habeas corpus was recognized as often frivolous. Time and again, a new dodge would appear, a writ would be taken, and years would pass. Any argument was useful. For example, when a black was sentenced to death, the objection of jury discrimination was regularly urged, even when the trial was eminently fair and the black defendant in fact would not have wanted blacks sitting on the jury. In one case in California, not especially unusual, there were eight trials, costing the State over $500,000.

When court procedures are finally exhausted, when review is no longer pending, the fate of the prisoner passes into the hands of the executive branch of the government which, under the United States system, is charged with carrying out or executing the orders of the judiciary. It has been generally assumed that the jury's decision imposing the death penalty was carried out—at least following appeals. But what actually happened at this stage?

In many jurisdictions, the governor had to order the execution, and he often avoided the decision as long as possible. Reprieves were commonplace. He could, definitively, avoid the execution by pardon or by commutation of the death sentence to a prison term. Governors often hesitated to intervene in this way, however, because they felt they would be usurping the power of the court. Twelve jurors—not the governor—listened at the trial. Interposition often occurred in another way.

The warden (or sheriff) having custody of the prisoner plays a principal role in the implementation of the penalty. The execution of the penalty depends very much on the attitude of the warden toward the penalty. The criminal law has three concepts of incapacity (insanity), each pertinent to a different stage: the capacity to stand trial, the capacity to commit crime, and the capacity to be executed under a death warrant. In the majority of states, the issue of postconviction insanity may be raised only by the warden.

The Supreme Court has never ruled that the Constitution precludes a state from executing a man who has temporarily or permanently become insane, but the rule has been well established either by statute or common law, although the logic behind the rule is vague. In the words of one jurist, "Whatever the reason of the law is, it is plain the law is so." One might argue that if anyone is to be executed it should be the criminally insane. One judge, dissenting against the rule, said: "Is it not an inverted humanitarianism that deplores as barbarous the capital punishment of those who have become insane after trial and conviction but accepts the capital punishment of sane men?"

Explanations for the exemption rule, as found in the literature, are various. It is said: "If the defendant is sane he might urge some reason not previously considered why the sentence should not be carried out." This theory offers the condemned man a last chance to prove his innocence. Yet the same logic would suffice to postpone, perhaps indefinitely, the execution of a sane man; for time for intelligent reflection may disclose new reasons for stay of execution of the sane as well. To quote another explanation: "Killing an insane person does not have the same moral quality as killing a sane person." The moral basis underlying the forensic responsibility rule at the time of the deed is carried over until the time of execution, although the person was found legally sane and responsible at the time of the deed. A third defense of the rule involves the conception of the self. God would not, on the Great Day, make a person answer for that of which he remembered nothing: he is not the same person. The law likewise says that a man is not subject to execution for crime when "he is not the same person forensically now which he was then." But, as Heraclitus long ago explained, all is flux. It may be noted that supervening insanity, although cause to interrupt an appeal or stay an execution, does not suspend a prison term. A convict who turns insane in prison may be transferred to the security unit of a mental institution; but this rarely happens, because conditions in the criminal insane section of the hospital are pitiful in comparison to conditions at the prison. In the event of transfer, time spent in the mental institution is credited toward the prison sentence. Finally, some insist that the rule is based on the lack of retributory satisfaction derived by society in executing an insane person. A related belief is that "a person should not be put to death while insane because in that condition he is unable to make his peace with God." To a modern audience, this argument is hardly convincing, and the condemned man himself often rejects spiritual solace in his final hours and looks instead to a good last meal.

Whatever the underlying reasons, however illogical they may be, the rule has been perpetuated, either by statute or judicial decision, in every state having the death penalty. However, the procedure by which the rule is implemented is slipshod. At common law the prisoner was brought before a judge who either decided the question of insanity himself or at his discretion impaneled a jury to assist him. A few states have retained this or a similar procedure. But most states in practice, if not in law, have entrusted the initial decision to a prison or police official.

The Supreme Court, in 1950 in *Solesbee v. Balkom*, said that postponement of execution because of postconviction insanity bears a close affinity not to trial but to reprieves of sentences, which is an executive power, and "seldom, if ever, has this power of executive clemency been subjected to review by the courts."[2] In the *Solesbee* case the Court found that Georgia had not violated due process in constituting its governor an "apt and special tribunal" for determining, in ex parte proceedings, the sanity of a condemned man at the time of execution. (In federal and military cases, Lincoln was apparently the first President to intercede in an execution on account of supervening insanity.)

The inquiry may be entirely behind closed doors without any opportunity for submission of facts on behalf of the person whose sanity is to be determined. It has long been recognized that due process does not require that a condemned man who asserts supervening insanity be given a full judicial proceeding to adjudicate his claim. In 1897, in *Nobles v. Georgia*, the Supreme Court said that if such proceedings were required "it would be wholly at the will of a convict to suffer any punishment whatever, for the necessity of his doing so would depend solely upon his fecundity in making suggestion after suggestion of insanity, to be followed by trial upon trial."[3]

In *Solesbee*, the Supreme Court, noting that the governor in deciding on execution had the aid of specifically trained physicians, went on to say:

It is true that governors and physicians might make errors of judgment. But the search for truth in this field is always beset by difficulties that may beget error. Even judicial determination of sanity might be wrong. . . . We cannot say that it offends due process to leave the question of a convicted person's sanity to the solemn responsibility of a state's highest executive with authority to invoke the aid of the most skillful class of experts on the crucial questions involved.

In this case, the condemned man lost out, but if the governor decides in his favor, a fortiori, no one is interested or has standing to complain to the courts.

The power of the governor is often delegated to agencies such as pardon and parole boards. In 1958, in *Caritativo v. California*, the Court, extending its decision in *Solesbee*, upheld a procedure whereby the initiation of proceedings to determine the sanity of a condemned man in his custody is made by the warden in his sole judgment.[4] If the warden "has good reason to believe" that a condemned man has become insane, he must so advise the judge or district attorney of the judicial district where the convict was sentenced, and an investigation may be ordered. If the warden does not take the first step, no judge or officer other than the governor can suspend the execution of a death sentence. The condemned man is given no right to commence a judicial or any other type of proceeding.

Justice Harlan, in *Caritativo*, said: "Surely it is not inappropriate for [the state] to lodge this grave responsibility in the hands of the warden, the official who beyond all others had had the most intimate relations with, and best opportunity to observe, the prisoner." But Justice Frankfurter, joined by Justices Brennan and Douglas, strongly dissented:

Now it appears that [the determination of the sanity of a man condemned to death], upon which depends the fearful question of life or death, may . . . be made on the mere say-so of the warden of a state prison, according to such procedure as he chooses to pursue, and more particularly without any right on the part of a man awaiting death who claims that insanity has supervened to have his case put to the warden. There can hardly be a comparable situation under our constitutional scheme of things in which an interest so great, that an insane man not be executed, is given such flimsy procedural protection and where one asserting a claim is denied the rudimentary right of having his side submitted to the one who sits in judgment.

A person under death sentence is sentenced to death; he is not sentenced to prison. He is placed under the custody of the warden. He is not part of the prison population. He is placed in a separate cell. In the United States, where legal maneuvers in capital cases usually take several years, the prisoner during this time sits in isolation on death row. Earlier, during the trial stage, which rarely takes less than a year, he sat in jail, without opportunity for release on bail, and usually without therapy. Following conviction, death even more preys on his mind. In the words of one prisoner: "The days are so long. There is nothing to pass the time. Nothing to keep your mind occupied. I feel like I don't even exist. I'm here and I'm not here. I have headaches. I just want to scream."

Wait long enough and the prisoner will hallucinate (or he will die a natural death). He will deteriorate. Psychiatrists point out that offenders are usually people who release tension by acting out, by using muscle, and they become very anxious when locked up. Without any activity, they invariably break down and become psychotic. They explode into pieces. Capital offenders are likely to be unstable anyway, but solitary confinement does much to break down the sanity of the most normal of men, as the experiments of Hebb and others on sensory deprivation have vividly demonstrated. Governor Earl Long once remarked, "Who in hell wouldn't go mad?" (Louisiana at the time of the remark had not carried out an execution in over ten years.)[5]

If the condemned man does not become genuinely psychotic, he will find it expedient to malinger. He jumps up and down. He seldom does anything correctly. He makes absurd statements. When shown a watch reading 2:30 he may say the time is 6 o'clock. When shown a fifty-cent piece, he may call it a dollar bill. Such symptoms are popularly called the *nonsense syndrome,* and in psychiatry, the *Ganser syndrome.* The condemned man learns, either through the grapevine or from the subtle advice of his attorney, that under the law insanity precludes execution. As a last-ditch measure he may act upon this information. The condemned man is entitled to the information, just as a businessman has a right to advice on loopholes in the tax laws.

The following conversation, tape recorded, illustrates the contrivance which has been put on in the prison to effect transfer to the hospital.

EXAMINER AT HOSPITAL: Tell me what happened at the penitentiary to make them send you to the hospital.
PATIENT (FORMERLY PRISONER): Nothing.
EXAMINER: Huh?
PATIENT: My lawyer came and got me.
EXAMINER: Your lawyer came and got you? Are you afraid of dying?
PATIENT: (No answer.)
EXAMINER: Did your lawyer tell you what to do to get out of there?
PATIENT: No.
EXAMINER: Looks to me like a good lawyer would have told you how to act. He didn't tell you how to act?
PATIENT: (Inaudible mumbles.)
EXAMINER: I didn't understand you. He told you to act crazy?
PATIENT: Uh-hum.
EXAMINER: What did he say?
PATIENT: He kept telling me . . . (Inaudible).
EXAMINER: The last time he came up, what did he do?
PATIENT: He asked if I ever had an epileptic fit.
EXAMINER: What did you tell him?
PATIENT: I told him no.
EXAMINER: What did he say then?
PATIENT: He said that an epileptic fit was the last straw. (In the lingo, an epileptic fit is the way of a crazy man.)
EXAMINER: He told you this?
PATIENT: Yes.
EXAMINER: Did he tell you how to act?
PATIENT: No, he didn't want to incriminate himself.
EXAMINER: He told you that he did not want to incriminate himself?
PATIENT: That's right.
EXAMINER: So he didn't tell you how to act. But he got his point across to you?
PATIENT: (Inaudible.)
EXAMINER: Huh? How did you know how to act when he told you about epileptic fits?
PATIENT: I just knew.

Sporadic malingering is difficult to prove especially when the motivation to fake is great. In the prison setting, however, as Justice Harlan noted, the individual may be observed on a twenty-four-hour basis; over this period of time it is difficult to keep up a simulated psychosis. Prison personnel can usually spot an inmate whose bizarre behavior is an act. They know "he's not a real psycho." The problem becomes more difficult when an unstable person begins to fake mental illness, and then, like a man running downhill, finds he cannot stop.

Happily for the condemned man, prison officials in most states have usually closed their eyes to the simulation. Who wants to pull the switch? The condemned man's keepers get to know him, and they develop some feeling for him. As they dislike executing anyone, they have tended to accept feigned craziness as genuine. So, ostensibly for observation or treatment, the condemned man has been referred to a prison psychiatrist or transferred to the security area of a mental hospital (the criminal insane section) where he usually has lived out the rest of his days, often as a trusty.

One easily believes what one wishes to believe. Wardens and psychiatrists, perhaps for different reasons, can readily find a symptom of madness. There is always evidence available, however episodic, to warrant a stay of execution. The Supreme Court has conceded, "The search for truth in this field is always beset by difficulties that may beget error." The law has long recognized that people may have lucid intervals and nonlucid intervals. Psychiatrists use labels such as *dissociative states* and *three-day schizophrenia*. We are disintegrated when we wake up in the morning and when we are asleep. "We pull ourselves together." We all have "crazy spells." We question at times the judgment of our best friends and colleagues, and at such times we call them crazy. It is not possible to have a touch of pregnancy, but it is possible to have a touch of psychosis; the latter is not an all-or-none condition. Part of one's personality may be affected by a psychotic process, but the remnants of the ego may function properly. Given the type of person who commits a capital crime, mental and emotional aberrations of marked degree are readily in evidence. There is also the syndrome in which the prisoner thinks he is malingering, and the warden or psychiatrist knows the prisoner thinks so, but justifiably considers him crazy nonetheless.

There is a direct corollary between the number and the location of executions. The execution of the death penalty has depended to a marked degree on whether the chair is moved around from jailhouse to jailhouse or whether all condemned persons are sent to a centralized place—the state penitentiary—for execution. During the past twenty or thirty years many states have enacted legislation providing that executions are to be carried out at the state penitentiary rather than at the various county jails. Legislators, possessing the ability to see problems in both ideological and financial terms, realize it is expensive and cumbersome to transport the chair from jail to jail.

When execution of the death penalty is to take place in the local or county jail, it is more likely to be carried out. For one reason, the condemned man, when in the state penitentiary, far removed from the scene of the crime, is more likely to be forgotten by an enraged community than if he remained in close proximity to the scene of the crime. For another, the warden of a penitentiary is in a position very different from that of the sheriff of a local jailhouse. The warden is practically a feudal lord, and his attitude is likely to be every bit as imperious. He feels the inherent power of his position, and he is usually willing to exercise the broad discretion to postpone invested in him by law.

In former times it was customary for an execution to take place as near as possible to the scene of the crime. A nearby tree was selected or a gallows was erected in a large open space in the town. By the 1930s, with a few exceptions, public executions disappeared from the American scene. Citizens organized to prohibit public executions because, as reports in newspapers of the time disclose, "the crowds often assumed the characteristics of a mob and often indulged in the wildest and most unrestrained orgies." The executions incited widespread agitation, brawling, drunkenness, and crime. Many good citizens got carried away in the heat and violence of the moment and participated in some dreadful acts. So executions were first moved from outdoors to inside the local jailhouse, and then gradually, as noted, from the local jailhouse to the state penitentiary. But what happened there?

The population of the state penitentiary is large, and the atmosphere there is ordinarily tense. It becomes volatile whenever there is an execution. The macabre event provokes brawling and violence among the convicts, as it formerly did on the outside among the citizenry. The warden is motivated to defer the execution not only because he has some feelings for the condemned man but also because he values his job. All administrators want things to run smoothly. Unpleasant publicity is the bane of officialdom; and riots make ugly headlines.

But headlines of a different nature may exert influence on the warden in the other direction. The more publicity attending the trial, the more famous or notorious the criminal, the more likely the execution. In such cases, the warden rarely "has good reason to believe" that the prisoner has become insane, and he finds it expedient not to initiate an investigation. Fredric Wertham, psychiatrist and writer, was denied permission to see Ethel Rosenberg when she was at Sing Sing; but in earlier interviews her attorney reported her as in despair, without lipstick or makeup, her hair uncombed, "not caring how she looked." In Kansas, a young man, Lee Andrews, was sentenced to death for the murder of his parents. He was a university student and spent his time in his cell reading books. He did not act crazy. In addition, prominent citizens intervened asking executive clemency, much to the annoyance of the governor. The case was headlined in the papers. As a result, widespread attention focused on Andrews, and he was executed. California regularly executes its condemned men (following a protracted and expensive judicial process), but even outside California, Caryl Chessman probably would have been executed. The eyes of the world were upon him. Ironically, he protested too much. He made too much noise, and he protested via book-writing—the mark of a rational man.

In *Caritativo*, it was held proper for the state to condition a condemned man's right to a sanity investigation upon a preliminary determination by the warden that "good reason exists for the belief that the convict has become insane." More often than not, the various reasons underlying the rule of "competency to be executed" merge or fade away into the simple statement, "you're not supposed to execute someone who doesn't know what's happening." Theoretically, mental illness, of itself, is not sufficient to bring into operation the rule of suspension of execution. Mental illness as a legal concept is not identical with the medical concept of the term. It may be that a person who does not know what is happening is mentally ill, but mental illness alone is not the test. Indeed, a person may be mentally well but nonetheless may not know what is happening, for example, a person of very low intelligence.

Actually, the test on executionability is meaningless. It would not even exempt the blithering idiot. In several recent rulings the Supreme Court made no reference to the reasons for the rule but simply said, in dictum, that it is unlawful to execute a prisoner who has become insane after his conviction. Theory notwithstanding, medical status of itself thus serves as a haven from legal action.

Although the Supreme Court in *Caritativo* specifically stated that wardens are not obliged to obtain a psychiatric examination of the condemned man, they have as a general practice delegated the responsibility to a prison psychiatrist, or, with the authorization of the trial court, have transferred him to the security treatment area of a mental hospital for examination and treatment. In this way, the warden guarantees "a responsible and good-faith determination," and he is usually satisfied with the result. The trial court invariably will postpone execution, without date, when it receives a psychiatric report stating that the condemned man does not realize he is to be executed for the crime he has committed.

To review, the jury—a group so large that individual responsibility is lost—relieves the judge of the death-penalty decision at the trial. The judge then transfers the condemned man to the warden who is able to delegate the responsibility to the psychiatrist. Thus, in the end, the decision on execution of the death penalty is left to one individual—the psychiatrist. He is given a nonmedical—and absurd—responsibility. He is asked to report back to the warden when "this man is ready to be electrocuted."

Professor Albert Ehrenzweig, of the University of California Law School, compares the procedure to a game of ping-pong, but this is hardly an apt comparison. The psychiatrist knows that the warden does not want him to make a return play. He rarely reports that his patient, regardless of his mental status, is "ready to be electrocuted," although, as a matter of fact, in this age of tranquilizing drugs a man could readily be shaped up for execution.

While death may be postponed for the condemned man while in the security treatment unit, his stay there does not always encourage forgetfulness of his sentence. With inadequate facilities, attendants, and security protection, mental hospitals find discipline a stiff problem in these units. Consequently, prisoners transferred from the penitentiary to the hospital are warned that misbehavior will result in their being sent back "to fry." The capital-penalty abolitionist may take note that, here, recalcitrant persons already condemned to death can be deterred by the threat of execution. Every now and then, the hospital director, to show he means business, returns an unruly inmate to the penitentiary—and to his death. This accounts for many of the executions in states where, according to statistics, they occur sporadically.

Another punitive practice in the security treatment unit of many hospitals involves the conversion of electroshock treatment (EST) from a therapy to a threat. In ordinary psychiatric practice, EST is the somatic therapy of choice in cases of depression. Its potential as a punishment, however, is obvious: a little electricity cures, but it hurts, and too much kills. Furthermore, for a man facing the electric chair, the psychological implications in the threat of being "buzzed" can well be imagined.

None of these unpleasant procedures for controlling the condemned man in the hospital's security area, however, seem half as bizarre on close look as authority's reason for putting him there. The psychiatrist is asked to *treat* the prisoner (patient). To what end? Why, so that he may be electrocuted! This goal of therapy is, indeed, a curious footnote to the Hippocratic oath. Little wonder that the psychiatrist, with a prisoner on his hands who has been brought out of his psychotic state by EST or drugs, fails to report that the man is "ready to be electrocuted!" The psychiatrist knows that such a statement from him is tantamount to an endorsement of the death penalty, so he is likely to play it cool and do nothing or use delaying tactics. Ordinarily, he is not in sympathy with the death penalty; but, in any event, he feels that the decision is not for him to make. "Who is fit to be executed?" is a moral, not a scientific inquiry. Society cannot fairly blame the psychiatrist for taking the law into his own hands. As Menninger says: "Most psychiatrists dislike very much being called in when somebody wants to know if the accused is well enough so that his head may be chopped off. I don't think the psychiatrist is very interested in acting as assistant to the executioner." Clearly, psychiatrists share the understandable human trait of being reluctant to push a person down the road to death. Moreover, they are doctors whose training and credo aim to preserve life, not to hasten its ending. Their attitude toward the condemned man as patient is readily explained.

But what about the law—the law of the land—that shall prevail? How do we explain this reluctance, this dalliance and indecision that has marked the course of the law all along the way from death sentence to death row? Although the ultimate-punishment issue has evoked national debate for at least a century and a half, it is clear that by a cumbersome and slipshod method, the penalty was in effect eliminated long before the Supreme Court's decision in 1972 voiding jury discrimination in sentencing.

The method has historical antecedents and is commonplace. Moral issues are often turned into medical decisions. Historically, for example, individuals were rescued from persecution by the Church with the introduction of a medical assumption: "The people are not possessed by the devil or by demons; they are sick. . . . They are not witches and therefore should not be burnt at the stake."

The capacity-to-stand-execution procedure, via the executive department, achieved the functional abolition of the death penalty. The repugnance felt for the death penalty emerged cloaked as a rational medical decision. Perhaps this was not a chance achievement.

NOTES

1. The Court ruled in three cases, all involving black defendants, one of them for a robbery-murder, and two for rape. *Furman v. Georgia,* 408 U.S. 238 (1972). The death penalty is on the statute books of all states except fourteen—Alaska, Hawaii, Iowa, Maine, Michigan, Minnesota, New Mexico, New York, North Dakota, Oregon, Rhode Island, Vermont, West Virginia, and Wisconsin. In California and New Jersey, the state supreme courts had ruled that capital punishment was unconstitutional. The history of the recent abolitionist movement is related in Meltsner, M. *Cruel and Unusual: The Supreme Court and Capital Punishment.* New York: Random House, 1973.
2. 339 U.S. 9 (1950).
3. 168 U.S. 398 (1897).
4. 357 U.S. 549 (1958).
5. Gallemore, J. L., and Panton, J. H. Inmate Responses to Lengthy Death Row Confinement. *Am. J. Psychiatry* 129:167, 1972.

8. The Psychiatric Court Clinic

"L ET the punishment fit the crime" is a cliché learned as children from Gilbert and Sullivan; and at one time it was the byword of major penal reform. Proponents of this principle in England sought to limit the application of the death penalty, which was exacted for over 160 offenses, on the ground that such a harsh penalty did not fit all these offenses.

Modern-day reformers advocate an individualized approach in which the punishment must fit the criminal, not simply the crime. Themis, the ancient Greek goddess of justice and equity, was once depicted with large, wide-open eyes, but since the late nineteenth century, she has been blindfolded, emphasizing the objectivity or anonymity with which justice is meted out. Emphasis on the act was an important political achievement, assuring equality before the law. A criminal act was to be adjudged and punished the same, at least that was the hope, whether committed by a prince or a pauper. Reformers would now have Themis remove her blindfold and look at the actor as well as the act— not at whether the actor is a prince or pauper but at the psychodynamics of the actor's behavior.

Frequently, the policeman ("the court of first instance") is the only one who considers both the act and the actor. The officer who makes the arrest sees the accused and perhaps talks with him. After being booked in the precinct station, however, the accused becomes more a number than a person as he is processed through the various stages of the criminal proceeding. The accused is prosecuted, tried, and processed depending upon the type of offense committed. Offenses are generally divided into four classes: class one (e.g., murder, rape), punishable by death or life imprisonment; class two (e.g., armed robbery, burglary), punishable by imprisonment at hard labor; class three (e.g., theft over $100, pandering, crime against nature), punishable by imprisonment with or without hard labor; and class four (e.g., simple battery, prostitution), punishable by fine or imprisonment.

In medicine, the physician considers the medical history of the patient. In law, on the other hand, evidence of the defendant's prior acts is inadmissible to prove guilt as the defendant is not obliged to defend his life history. As a general proposition, a defendant's prior difficulties with the law, such as specific prior criminal acts or bad reputation, cannot be used by the prosecutor even though such facts might tend to prove a defendant's propensity to commit the crime for which he is on trial.

Speaking on the inadmissibility of evidence of bad character to establish a probability of guilt, the Supreme Court has stated:

> Not that the law invests the defendant with a presumption of good character . . . but it simply closes the whole matter of character, disposition, and reputation on the prosecution's case-in-chief. The state may not show defendant's prior trouble with the law, specific criminal acts, or ill name among his neighbors, even though such facts might logically be persuasive that he is by propensity a probable perpetrator of the crime. The inquiry is not rejected because character is irrelevant; on the contrary, it is said to weigh too much with the jury and to so overpersuade them as to prejudge one with a bad general record and deny him a fair opportunity to defend against a particular charge. The overriding policy of excluding such evidence, despite its admitted probative value, is the practical experience that its disallowance tends to prevent confusion of issues, unfair surprise, and undue prejudice.[1]

What about beyond proof of guilt? The criminal law's approach of looking to the act rather than to the actor, if literally applied, is mechanical. It has been suggested that the law of the act and that of the actor can be compromised by a dual-track approach, that is, by proceeding on the basis of the act at the trial level and on the basis of the actor at the sentencing and postsentencing levels. Regarding the sentence determination, the Supreme Court recently observed that "it is surely true that a trial judge generally has wide discretion" and "before making that determination, a judge may appropriately conduct an inquiry broad in scope, largely unlimited either as to the kind of information he may consider, or the source from which it may come."[2]

Toward the end of the nineteenth century, legislatures began to announce that the basic purpose of the criminal law was correction or rehabilitation rather than punishment. It was an endorsement of various declarations. The Declaration of Principles adopted by the first congress of the American Prison Association in 1870 said, "[T]reatment is directed to the criminal rather than to the crime, [hence] its great object should be his moral regeneration . . . not the infliction of vindictive suffering." The declaration called for classification of criminals "based on character"; for the indeterminate sentence under which the offender would be released as soon as the "moral cure" had been effected and "satisfactory proof of reformation" obtained; for "preventive institutions for the reception and treatment of children not yet criminal but in danger of becoming so"; for education as a "vital force in the reformation of fallen men and women"; and for prisons of a moderate size, preferably designed to house no more than three hundred inmates.

The Wickersham Commission, appointed by President Hoover in 1931, stated in its report:

We conclude that the present prison system is antiquated and inefficient. It does not reform the criminal. It fails to protect society. There is reason to believe that it contributes to the increase of crime by hardening the prisoner. We are convinced that a new type of penal institution must be developed, one that is new in spirit, in method, and in objective. The Commission recommends: individual treatment . . . indeterminate sentence . . . education in the broadest sense . . . skillful and sympathetic supervision of the prisoner on parole . . .

Two committees, one representing the American Bar Association and the other the American Psychiatric Association, met in 1929 to draft a position statement which advocated:

1. That there be available to every criminal and juvenile court a psychiatric service to assist the court in the disposition of offenders.

2. That no criminal be sentenced for any felony in any case in which the judge has any discretion as to the sentence until there be filed as a part of the record a psychiatric report.

3. That there be a psychiatric service available to each penal and correctional institution.

4. That there be a psychiatric report on every prisoner convicted of a felony before he is released.

5. That there be established in every state a complete system of administrative transfer and parole and that there be no decision for or against any parole or any transfer from one institution to another without a psychiatric report.

Thereafter, representatives of the APA and the ABA met with members of the American Medical Association, and the same recommendations were unanimously endorsed by the latter group. Thus official bodies of psychiatrists, physicians, and lawyers of the United States were in agreement on these principles, although in practice they have been largely ignored.

Under the law the prosecutor is not entitled to interview or examine the accused but must make out his case on the basis of evidence presented by others. The proposals of the ABA and APA of 1929 would not tamper with this traditional limitation on the prosecutor. Generally, it is only when a plea of insanity, incompetency to stand trial, or a sexual psychopath statute is at issue that a commission is appointed by the court to examine the defendant. The goal of the recommended principles is to make psychiatric services available to the court or institution in other instances as well.

Whether all lawbreakers should be dealt with in the same way, depending only on their offense, or whether physical and mental conditions should be given relevance are questions which must be agreed upon initially if the proposals are to become meaningful. Should a man who has a peptic ulcer be dealt with differently from a man not so afflicted? Should a woman who is manifestly depressed be handled differently from a woman who presents no visible signs of depression? Should a stupid individual be dealt with differently from an openly hostile one? Traditionally the law gives relevance only to minority and insanity (as defined by the M'Naughten or Durham test) in personalizing an offense.

On the one hand, it is argued that individualization of disposition would result in a rule of men replacing a rule of law. The basic meaning of *law*, it is said, is holding all men responsible to the same rules. The law, through its representatives in the courts and prisons, it is argued, has no business concerning itself with the whole person but only with that person's unlawful acts. When the whole person is considered, irrelevant factors or arbitrariness are more apt to enter the picture. If the whole person is to be considered, what will be looked for? The street gang in *West Side Story* pleaded, "Gee, Officer Krupke, deep down inside there is good!"

In a report, *Struggle for Justice: A Report on Crime and Punishment in America*, prepared for the Society of Friends and published in 1971, the American Friends Service Committee contends that the basic principle underlying the rule of law has been lost in recent decades as the shifting focus of the criminal system from the act to the individual gave rise to the practice of varying criminal sanctions according to individual characteristics. There being no sound scientific or moral basis for such variations, the Report strongly recommends a return to the principle of uniform application of penal sanctions. It is felt that society should have a limited set of rules stating which types of behavior are not permissible, that these rules should apply to absolutely everybody, and that they should be enforced with absolute consistency. The Report would replace the Department of Corrections, which it considers a euphemism, by a Department of Punishment. The recommendation is that all treatment be made voluntary. (Hegel contended that a criminal "does not receive his due honor unless the concept and measure of his punishment are derived from his own act" and "still less does he receive it if he is treated either as a harmful animal who has to be made harmless or with a view to deterring or reforming him.")

It is not clear how much change is actually proposed in the Report, since the committee presently sees no alternatives to prisons, feels that second offenses should be punished with increased severity, and would retain the chief features of indeterminacy, such as good time, though subject to judicial appeal. Its argument in favor of "uniformly distributing punishment according to what the act calls for" (whatever that means) fails to address itself to the fact that de jure equality usually results in de facto inequality. Is there not merit in discrimination when the individualization is done on a rational rather than arbitrary basis? If discretion were to play no role in the judicial process, then machines could replace judge or jury.

An individual commits a heinous act. Should he be sent to a hospital or to prison? Is he ill rather than bad? Is he able to control his hostile urges? Should he be afforded counseling or supervision? Should he be given medication? If certain individuals should not be incarcerated, why put them through the criminal law process at all? The psychiatric evaluation of offenders is premised on a philosophy of individualized processing.

Four cases may serve as illustration. Should these persons have been left alone, processed through the criminal law, or sent to a hospital? In these cases focus was placed on the offense rather than on the offender, consequently they were handled through the process of the criminal law.

1. Merle Survive killed his mother, and then proceeded to have sexual relations with her dead body. He was charged with first-degree murder.

2. Ethel Bailey, a middle-aged woman, was charged with aggravated arson. She set fire to the mattress in her rented house "to destroy the evil spirits" and sat there with her four-year-old son until the firemen arrived.

3. Botsford Sump was charged with burglary. He had been involved in two similar incidents before in which he broke into a home and would simply stand over a bed occupied by a female. At the time of the incident he was seeing a psychiatrist who reported that he had been working with him and that he seemed to be doing fine. He had a job and re-

portedly was getting along well with his wife and children. His lawyer, attempting to have the charge dismissed, said, "A man who enters a house and looks down at a woman in bed and has done so on three occasions is a sick man and not a burglar. Labeling a man a criminal, when in reality he is sick and can be cured, is a disservice to society. The man who is labeled a criminal has difficulty obtaining work and supporting a family and the repercussions are catastrophic." The district attorney, however, was mindful of adverse publicity in the press and refused to dismiss the case at that point. He might have refused the charge initially, however, if he had been sure the individual would be put in a hospital.

4. Hedy Lamarr allegedly shoplifted about $86 worth of goods. At the time she was carrying $14,000 in royalty checks in her pocketbook. She said, at the time of her arrest, "I am willing to pay for these things. Other stores let me do it." Harry Golden, commenting on the case, said:

Whoever arrested Hedy Lamarr was a particularly consciousless and/or stupid store detective. Every store employs detectives to step up to a kleptomaniac and whisper, "Now please pay the cashier." When as a reporter, I went around to stores years ago on a feature story about shoplifting, I found the system was even then decades old. The eagle-eye toted up what the shoplifter took, and if she couldn't pony up the money, the store manager called her father or husband and recited the amount owed and the father or husband always said, "I'll put a check in the mail immediately." Then the woman went to a psychiatrist and I have discovered that in this one particular area, psychiatry works wonders. Of course, we are not discussing thieves who make off with thousands of dollars of merchandise, or those who deal in stolen goods. This is a police matter and not a case for a psychiatrist. Any store detective worth his or her salt can tell the difference between a kleptomaniac and a thief. Any store detective who doesn't recognize Hedy Lamarr and know she has this problem, and further know she is good for the merchandise, ought to be hawking peanuts and not at Shea Stadium in New York but at the big league ball park in Milwaukee.[3]

At the trial Hedy Lamarr's son testified that she had been distressed the day she was arrested because, among other things, "she was not as beautiful as she had been." A psychiatrist testified that he did not think she could have formulated the intent to deprive the store of the property as she was under emotional stress. She was acquitted.[4]

A judge once remarked that the primary function of a jury is not to determine guilt or innocence—that would be too easy a task—but rather to decide what should be done with the defendant. Lawyers experienced in the practice of criminal law commonly say that no less than 98 percent of defendants who come before the courts are in fact guilty. The judge or jury looks at the defendant and at the complaining witness, compares them, and decides accordingly. Perhaps the cases just described were properly dealt with, perhaps not. In any event the decisions were not made after full exploration. These cases all occurred within days of each other, over fifty years after the establishment of the first adult court psychiatric clinic.

The concept of a court clinic or diagnostic center had its origin in 1909 when William Healy began his pioneer work in Cook County Juvenile Court in Chicago.[5] This led to the establishment of the Psychopathic Laboratory, the first adult court psychiatric clinic, in the same city in 1914. The idea did not spread as rapidly as many of its advocates had expected. At first, the idea spread quickly, and in the early 1920s clinics were established either informally or by legislative act in a number of cities. However, the trend lagged during the war and postwar years.

The organization and operation of the clinics which now exist are by no means uniform. The variety represents, to some degree, the different philosophies of the legal and psychiatric professions as to the method whereby such service should be integrated into the administration of the criminal law.[6] The operation of the clinic, however, can be subsumed in either one or more of the following categories:

1. To conduct pretrial examinations to determine either the fitness of the defendant to stand trial or the legal responsibility of the defendant for the crime committed.

2. To conduct presentence examinations and prepare a report which the judge may use to determine the proper sentence or treatment for the offender.

3. To conduct postsentence examinations which may be for either of two purposes: preparation of a psychiatric history and recommendations for the treatment of the offender at the institution or penitentiary, to whichever he is sent; or recommendations as to the proper course of therapy to be followed, if needed, when the offender is placed on probation.

Each of these operations, which may be carried out by a court-appointed examiner as well as by a clinic, has its advantages and disadvantages. In the case of a pretrial examination, an evaluation may serve to keep the offender out of the criminal law process when it would serve no useful function. There is a practice of dismissing a charge if the accused will go to a psychiatrist for treatment, and if the psychiatrist will indicate that the accused is not a threat to himself or to others. Pretrial examination, however, is mainly performed with a view toward its use at trial. Through the efforts of Dr. Vernon L. Briggs, a law was passed in 1921 in Massachusetts which requires that every defendant charged with a felony be given a psychiatric examination prior to his trial and that the evidence be made available at the trial. Kentucky and Michigan subsequently enacted statutes comparable to the Briggs Law. Unfortunately in such a system, there is a tendency for the examinations to be made perfunctorily and in a disinterested fashion. Moreover, psychiatrists are often reluctant to participate in pretrial examinations because they will likely become involved as witnesses at trial, and they know that court appearances are time-consuming and cross-examinations often humiliating.

An example of a posttrial operation is the Kansas State Reception and Diagnostic Center, located near the Menninger Foundation and drawing upon its resources. Established in 1961 with Dr. Karl Menninger as its motivating force, its purpose is "to provide a thorough and scientific examination and study of all felony offenders of the male sex sentenced by the courts . . . to state penal institutions so that each such offender may be assigned to a state penal institution having the type of security (maximum, medium, or minimum) and programs of education, employment, or treatment designed to accomplish a maximum of rehabilitation for such offender."[7] In order to implement the purpose of the Center, which is concerned only with postsentence evaluation, Kansas enacted a law giving the trial judge the unusual authority to modify a sentence after its imposition, so as to take account of the Center's report.[8] The trial judge may modify a sentence within 120 days after its imposition to grant probation. Since the court can reduce but not increase the original sentence, following the Center's report, there is a tendency in initial sentencing to impose the maximum. The prisoner, who is sent to the Center for a maximum sixty-day period of evaluation, usually tries to con the examiner, putting on convincing acts of subservience. The cost of operation is approximately five times per man more costly than prison, a fact which some legislators find difficult to justify.

A postsentence examination often comes too late. By that time the offender has already been evaluated by the policeman, the district attorney, and the judge or jury. In effect, examination by the clinic is a fourth evaluation, and therefore it should come as no surprise that most of the recommendations made at this time suggest that the offender be kept in custody. Moreover, the type of person referred by the judge is usually one who is an annoyance to him (e.g., he may refer only bad-check writers). Initiation of the psychiatric examination is thus left to a person who is generally unfamiliar with the symptoms of mental disorders. Finally, it should be noted that recommendations which are made for the purpose of treatment of the offender in some penitentiary or institution are often fanciful. If the examining psychiatrist has no familiarity with the institution to which the individual will be sent, he is not in a position to make recommendations which can be realistically carried out.

A psychiatric court clinic's mode of operation is affected, at least in part, by its origin. For example, a clinic established as a result of community reaction to the occurrence of sexual crimes is likely to focus on such cases. A clinic created in a large measure due to demands from a committee on probation is likely to work through the probation department rather than directly with the court. The Detroit clinic, now defunct, showed a special interest in traffic offenders. In Maryland, where sentences are determinate, the Baltimore Clinic mainly carried out presentence examinations. The Center for Forensic Psychiatry in Ann Arbor, Michigan, essentially carries out only evaluations on competency to stand trial, although the legislation establishing the center authorized examinations at all stages of the criminal law process.

The makeup of the staff may differ according to the purpose of the clinic. Generally, however, the clinic is staffed by a combination of psychiatrists, psychologists, and often times social workers and correctional officers. These staff members, with differing viewpoints on the system of criminal justice, must work together as a team so that proper recommendations may be made to the court.

At most clinics, the staff is employed on a part-time basis. Because the clinics are publicly funded, adequate salaries are generally not available for full-time employment of competent personnel. This disadvantage is offset, in part, by the fact that a staff psychiatrist who works at the clinic on a part-time basis, while also engaging in general psychiatric work, has been found to have a better perspective while performing his work at the court clinic.

The actual work performed depends not only on the chief purpose of the clinic but also on the work load and the available personnel. In many clinics only a small proportion of cases get an exhaustive workup. The clinic's function is often to weed out the grossly abnormal, that is, the psychotic and the mental defective. The clinic's report generally estimates the patient's intelligence, describes any physical pathology present, and contains a personality evaluation. In many clinics the report will also contain a summary and recommendations as to the disposition to be made of the patient. Reports submitted to the court tend to be verbose, and as a consequence the judge often reads only the conclusional paragraph; Churchill during World War II limited all bureau reports made to him to one page. Treatment is not a function of most clinics. Those established more recently, however, often provide for talking or drug therapy while the offender is on probation, if the court finds this to be the best disposition to be made in a particular case.[9]

A different type of organization is the forensic psychiatric clinic such as the one established at Temple University which operated from 1965 to 1967 until it ran out of funds. At the earliest possible stage of a legal problem consultation was made available to indigents and their attorneys without fee. The reports were kept confidential by furnishing them to counsel, which brought them under the protection of the attorney-client privilege rather than under the much more limited physician-patient privilege. The services of the Temple clinic were unique, coming into operation at the earliest phase of the legal problem while the situation was still fluid and open. It was also unique in that its services were available for civil as well as criminal cases.[10] In the past, civil cases have been, for the most part, ignored in the operation of court clinics. Individuals often present themselves to legal agencies, however, with ostensible legal problems which mask or hide serious emotional problems. It may be merely happenstance that a person seeks a legal rather than a medical remedy.[11]

A forensic psychiatric clinic which has a university affiliation can play an important role in the education of medical students, law students, and probation officers. The affiliation also serves to overcome the difficulty of obtaining well-trained and competent psychiatrists. Too often, psychiatrists working in court clinics are unlicensed, poorly trained, and foreign-born, speaking poor English. It is particularly difficult to obtain competent psychiatrists to work in clinics which do not provide treatment. A further drawback is that psychiatrists who work exclusively in diagnostic and advisory clinics seem to lose their touch. In the court-clinic setting, a somewhat stereotyped image of the patient may emerge and cause a psychiatrist to lose perspective of his work. There is also the difficulty in attracting highly trained and scarce professional personnel because the public agency may be unable to pay adequate salaries. Affiliation with a university tends to overcome many of these obstacles.[12]

In litigation over a cow the court is told everything about the cow, but in litigation involving people, the court is told very little about them. In many jurisdictions computer technology has not been applied to police statistics, criminal identification, and crime records, and not even this information is available to deal with crime generally or with the offender in particular. The Honorable Sir Roger Ormrod, one of Her Majesty's Judges of the High Court of Justice, in an address at a recent Annual Conference of the Association of Law Teachers at the University of Sheffield stated:

I think it is true that in recent years, certainly since the war, courts are becoming more and more concerned with the individual person who is before them. In criminal cases we now try, very unsuccessfully very often, because the material and tools at our disposal are inadequate, and knowledge is inadequate, but we try to do something about the man individually. In the matrimonial field it is no longer enough to find somebody guilty of adultery, to say "the guilty party" and all the rest follows. Now the Court of Appeal has said and the new Act made it abundantly plain, that you have to consider the conduct of the parties as a whole. This means you have got to understand the interactions of the two personalities, one on the other, if you are to do anything remotely resembling justice. This is the individualisation of justice in its early stages. But it requires a great deal of new learning, new knowledge, on the part of lawyers. The old-fashioned type of submission, say in a custody case, making old hackneyed points does not help much when what you are really worrying about is what is this child like, what are his parents like, are they sympathetic, are they affectionate, is his father affectionate, or is the father trying to use the children to boost his own damaged ego, is the mother holding onto them because she has lost her husband and as a substitute, trying to make a boy into a substitute husband? Now I am only touching on this lightly, but these are the kinds of problem we now have to think about and we need help from the advocates. Transfer the scene into the criminal court and you listen to the speech in mitigation of the old-fashioned type—he is kind to his mother, he had, forty years ago, a distinguished war record, this kind of thing. What you want to know is why did this man do this? And what are we going to do with him? And have a sensible discussion backwards and forwards. I would like to hear the prosecution coming in on sentencing. I know this sounds like heresy, but why experienced advocates for the prosecution should sit there mum and do nothing but call the officer, and literally say "I will call the officer" and sit down while the record is read out, and give the court no assistance whatever as to what should be done with the man, I do not know. Here we have competent people on both sides who might have much more to contribute than to argue whether this piece of evidence is or is not admissible.[13]

Sentencing in the courts has become chaotic, with judges by their own account regularly handing out sentences they consider either too lenient or too harsh. A recent study by the *New York Times* found the following: (1) Unable to handle their case loads, courts and prosecutors allow a great deal of plea-bargaining, in which a defendant is offered a reduced charge and a light sentence in return for a guilty plea; (2) a loss of faith in the prison system by some judges which results in their refusal to send all but the most dangerous defendants to prison, and in cases where they do send a man to prison, they say, they do so unwillingly, believing they are creating an even worse criminal; and (3) a belief by some judges who say they knowingly give light sentences because sentences—whether light or harsh—do nothing to cut down crime.[14]

The sentencing crisis includes the problem of sentence disparities, i.e., of similar defendants, charged with similar crimes, getting vastly different sentences, reflecting differences in the defendant's finances, race, geography, and in the judge's personality. To many observers, sentences are determined with no precise guidelines. Some blame unfair sentences on the discretionary sentencing power invested in judges.

In response to the *Times* study, New York Chief Judge Stanley H. Fuld recommended the establishment of a special agency to study trial records and probation reports and then to make sentences on a consistent basis. The aim is not to achieve uniformity in sentencing—each defendant should be treated individually, dependent upon a myriad of considerations—but to avoid disparity in sentencing, where in generally similar situations, judges acting independently have sentenced with great variance. Judge Fuld said that the emphasis of the justice system should be shifted from "punishment to fit the crime" to "treatment to fit the offender." He stated:

Disparity in sentencing is most unfortunate. But, absent an intimate knowledge of (1) the evidence presented in the various cases, and (2) of the facts bearing up a particular defendant's past life, including his criminal record, it is impossible to assess intelligently the sentence imposed upon him, qualitatively or quantitatively, or to compare it with a sentence meted out to some other defendant.

To minimize disparity in sentencing, it may ultimately be demonstrated that it is desirable to commit to a correction authority or some other agency the responsibility and duty of determining the treatment to be accorded those convicted and to vest such agency with the power to determine whether the offender be placed on probation, be confined under conditions deemed to be in the public interest, to release him or parole him under such supervision and upon such conditions as it believes conducive to law-abiding conduct, or to discharge him when, in its judgment, further confinement or control is no longer required in the public interest.

I cannot refrain from repeating an observation which I made in the nineteen-forties, and have since frequently repeated, that an ideal criminal justice system would shift emphasis from prosecution to crime prevention, from the punishment of crime to the rehabilitative treatment of the offender; or, phrased somewhat differently, from the formula punishment to fit the crime, to the principle, treatment to fit the offender.

I recognize the unfortunate fact—as is the situation with all parts of the criminal justice system—that lack of funds has made it impossible to translate this ideal into practice. But, needless to say, we should not abandon our pursuit of that high aim.[15]

The forensic psychiatric clinic is an agency which could assist the court in obtaining a better idea of why a certain act was done, and to stimulate insight into the proper disposition that should be made of the offender. In getting at the cause of things and reaching a remedy, cartoonist Chon Day depicts one woman explaining her husband's newfound happiness, "First he was mad at the Republicans, then he was mad at the Democrats—then we found out his shoes were too tight." In a union of law and economics, Judge Charles Wyzanski, in the famous *United Shoe Machinery* case more than a decade ago, appointed a panel of leading economists to assist him as "law clerks" in understanding and dealing with economic competition. In a union of law and psychiatry, psychiatric court clinics assisting the court seem destined to multiply and expand, for it may be expected that many more offenders will be granted probation, sometimes conditioned upon psychiatric treatment. The American Bar Association in 1968 recommended that probation be preferred to prison where possible and that sentences for all but heinous crimes should generally not exceed five years.

The report of the President's Commission on Law Enforcement and Administration of Justice, entitled *The Challenge of Crime in a Free Society,* stated that procedures are needed to identify mentally disordered or deficient persons and to help officers who administer criminal justice to deal with them by means other than the ordinary criminal processes. The report concluded:

The Commission believes that, if any individual is to be given special therapeutic treatment, he should be diverted as soon as possible from the criminal process. It believes further that screening procedures capable of identifying mentally disordered or deficient offenders as early in the process as possible can be improved by training law enforcement and court officers to be more sensitive to signs of mental abormality by making specialized diagnostic referral services more readily available to the police and the court.

An evaluation, of course, is not the be-all and end-all. All the examinations in the world have only academic value unless they relate to something meaningful that will follow. Notwithstanding persuasive reasons, prisons have not been replaced by work camps. The McKay Commission in its report on the Attica prison rebellion said the "promise of rehabilitation" is but a "cruel joke."[16]

In general, a problem is more readily diagnosed than cured. Thus, the link is easy to establish between crime and slum-bred poverty, broken homes, rootlessness, availability of firearms, drugs, and limited police resources, but it is another matter to do something about them.

NOTES

1. *Michelson v. United States*, 335 U.S. 469 (1948).
2. *United States v. Tucker*, 92 S. Ct. 589, 591 (1972).
3. *Carolina Israelite*, Jan.–Feb. 1966, p. 13.
4. AP news release, April 23 and 26, 1966. In Arthur Hailey's account of the auto industry, one of the principal characters—a lonely, bored wife of an executive—shoplifts for the zest of it. Usually in such cases, if apprehended, the well-heeled make good the price and no criminal record is made. Hailey, A. *Wheels*. New York: Doubleday, 1971.
5. Psychiatry was and is used in the juvenile court in a flexible way relating to treatment considerations, but in the adult court it has been more commonly confined to questions such as criminal responsibility. The Institute for Juvenile Research was established as the Juvenile Psychopathic Institute to assist Judge Mary Bartelme of Chicago, the first judge of the first juvenile court in the United States. Established in 1909, the Institute was taken over by the county in 1913 and by the state in 1917. Sometime later the Commonwealth Foundation established demonstration clinics. A book by Helen L. Witmer on psychiatric clinics for children gives some interesting history. Witmer, H. L. *Psychiatric Clinics for Children*. New York: Commonwealth Fund, 1940.
6. Guttmacher, M. S.   Adult Psychiatric Court Clinics. In Slovenko, R. (Ed.). *Crime, Law and Corrections*. P. 479; see also Seligsohn, S.   Psychiatric Court Clinics. *Temp. L.Q.* 29:347, 1956.
7. *Kansas Stat. Ann.* 76-24a03. The Center is discussed in Targownik, K.   The Kansas State Reception and Diagnostic Center—Procedurally and Clinically. *Washburn L.J.* 6:285, 1967; Comment, The Kansas State Reception and Diagnostic Center: An Empirical Study. *Kan. L. Rev.* 19:821, 1971.
8. *Kansas Stat. Ann.* 62-2239.
9. O'Connell, B.   Court Clinics—The American Experience. *Med. Sci. & Law* 4: 266, 1964. The city court system of Baltimore and the University of Maryland Medical School recently established a special offenders clinic offering psychotherapy and supervision for non-violent sexual offenders and impulsively violent individuals. The program designers cited the need for such a facility in the face of the high recidivism rate for these offenders, whose problems have been "treated" with fines, imprisonment, or extended probation. *Psychiatr. News*, April 4, 1973, p. 20.
10. Sadoff, R. L., Polsky, S., and Heller, M. S.   The Forensic Psychiatry Clinic: Model for a New Approach. *Am. J. Psychiatry* 123:1402, 1967.
11. Modlin, H. C.   Sick or Bad? *Washburn L.J.* 6:307, 1967.
12. Guttmacher, M. S., *op. cit. supra* note 6.
13. Ormrod, R.   The Reform of Legal Education. *Law Teacher* 5:77, 1971.
14. *New York Times*, Sept. 26–27, 1972, p. 1.
15. *New York Times*, Sept. 28, 1972, p. 33.
16. In a film entitled, "Instead of Prison: Rehabilitating Offenders," Dr. Francis A. Tyce of the Minnesota State Hospital, Rochester, Minn., presents an innovative program for criminal offenders. Voluntarily residing in an open community facility, they make and enforce their own rules, vote new members in or out, take active part in constructive group discussions, and go to school, or work in the community. Roche Film Library, 600 Grand Ave., Ridgefield, N.J.